Textbook of
Neonatal Resuscitation

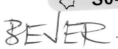

 American Heart Association

American Academy of Pediatrics

From an original text by
Ronald S. Bloom, MD, and
Catherine Cropley, RN, MN

Edited by Leon Chameides, MD,
and the AHA/AAP Neonatal
Resuscitation Steering Committee

© 1987, 1990 American Heart Association   ISBN 0-87493-605-5

American Heart Association
Committee on Emergency Cardiac Care, 1990—1991

Chairman

Richard E. Kerber, MD
Iowa City, Iowa

Members

Donald D. Brown, MD
Iowa City, Iowa

Richard O. Cummins, MD,
MPH, MSc
Seattle, Washington

Richard Melker, MD, PhD
Gainesville, Florida

Joseph P. Ornato, MD, FACC
Richmond, Virginia

James S. Seidel, MD, PhD
Torrance, California

American Heart Association
Subcommittee on Pediatric Resuscitation

Chairman

James S. Seidel, MD, PhD
Torrance, California

Members

J. Michael Dean, MD
Salt Lake City, Utah

Mary Fran Hazinski, MSN, RN
Nashville, Tennessee

Robert C. Luten, MD
Jacksonville, Florida

James M. McCrory, MD
Jacksonville, Florida

Olga Mohan, MD
Torrance, California

John R. Raye, MD
Farmington, Connecticut

Arno Zaritsky, MD
Chapel Hill, North Carolina

Neonatal Resuscitation Steering Committee
1990—1991

Cochairmen

William J. Keenan, MD
St. Louis, Missouri

John R. Raye, MD
Farmington, Connecticut

Members

Ronald S. Bloom, MD
Los Angeles, California

David Burchfield, MD
Gainesville, Florida

Consultants

Catherine Cropley, RN, MN
Culver City, California

Allen Erenberg, MD
Kansas City, Kansas

John Kattwinkel, MD
Charlottesville, Virginia

George J. Peckham, MD
Philadelphia, Pennsylvania

Preface

In the United States there are approximately 5,000 hospitals with delivery services in which about 3.7 million babies are born each year. Resuscitation is required for about 80% of the 30,000 babies with birth weights less than 1500 grams and for an unspecified additional number of those weighing more than 1500 grams at birth. Of the 5,000 hospitals, 90% are Level I institutions, 5% are Level II, and 5% are Level III facilities. Asphyxia continues to be a major neonatal problem, and neonatal resuscitation is frequently required in institutions without special neonatal expertise. This challenge was recognized both by the American Heart Association (AHA) and the American Academy of Pediatrics (AAP).

The Working Group on Pediatric Resuscitation, formed in 1978 under the auspices of the Emergency Cardiac Care Committee (ECC) of AHA, developed guidelines for neonatal resuscitation for the 1979 National Conference. A National Conference on Pediatric Resuscitation was convened in December, 1983 under the auspices of AHA, and one of the conclusions was that a training program for neonatal advanced life support was urgently needed. The guidelines for neonatal resuscitation were updated for the 1985 National Conference and endorsed by AAP. One of the stated goals was that "at least one person skilled in neonatal resuscitation should be in attendance at every delivery. An additional skilled person should be readily available. . . ."

The Section of Perinatal Pediatrics of AAP set up a task force in 1980 to investigate the need for a national program to teach infant resuscitation skills. Such a program was deemed necessary, was outlined and endorsed by the Executive Committee of AAP, and supported by representatives of the American College of Obstetrics and Gynecology, American Society of Anesthesiology, American Academy of Family Physicians, and the Canadian Pediatric Society.

This *Neonatal Resuscitation* course was the result of the combined efforts of the Working Group on Pediatric Resuscitation and the National Task Force on Neonatal Resuscitation of the Section on Perinatal Pediatrics of AAP. Its goal is to provide the materials and training necessary for health professionals in neonatal resuscitation according to AHA-AAP guidelines (*JAMA 1986; 255:2969—2973*). The original version by Ronald S. Bloom, MD, and Catherine Cropley, RN, MN, represented an extensive revision of a portion of the Neonatal Educational Program developed at the Charles R. Drew Postgraduate Medical School, under NHLBI-NIH contract N01-HR-5-2958. James Hand, PhD, Carl Hess, PhD, Marilyn Harz, MN, and Steven Westling, MA, were also involved in the development of the original program. This revision represents a consensus of the Neonatal Resuscitation Steering Committee.

Contents

Overview of the Program

The first moments of an infant's life can be critical. This is the time when the infant is making an abrupt transition from the mother's uterus to the extrauterine environment. A major problem that can arise during this time is asphyxia. Neonates are more often subject to asphyxia and are far more likely to be in need of resuscitation than any other age group. The way in which an asphyxiated infant is managed in the first few minutes of life can directly affect the quality of the individual's life and can have consequences over an entire lifetime.

Every newborn has a right to a resuscitation performed at a high level of competence. The proper equipment must be immediately available in the delivery room, and health care professionals must be skilled in resuscitating a newborn infant and capable of working smoothly as a team.

Lessons in the Program

As you go through this program, you will gain the knowledge and skills needed to perform neonatal resuscitation. The lessons described below contain the information needed to carry out the various components of the resuscitation procedure. Suggestions for using resuscitation equipment, manikins, and simulated situations for practice are included in the lessons. It is through such practice that you will attain the confidence and skill to perform a resuscitation correctly and in a timely manner.

The lessons comprising the entire program are as follows.

Lesson 1

Introduction to the Program

The first lesson introduces the program and provides the background information — key concepts, physiology elements of preparation, and some of the philosophy — that is helpful in approaching the resuscitation procedure effectively.

Lesson 2

Initial Steps in Resuscitation: Thermal Management, Positioning, Suctioning, and Tactile Stimulation

This lesson describes the first part of the resuscitation procedure and discusses the necessary steps in initially managing any infant immediately following delivery. Attention is given to the initial evaluation of the infant, decision making, and subsequent action based on the evaluation.

Lesson 3

Use of a Resuscitation Bag and Mask

Part A: Equipment
Part B: Ventilating the Infant
Part C: Ventilation as Part of the Resuscitation Procedure

This lesson has been divided into three parts. Part A introduces the equipment used for positive-pressure ventilation of an infant. Part B presents the fundamentals of using a resuscitation bag and mask. Part C describes the procedure in detail and deals with the key decisions that need to be made during the procedure.

Lesson 4   **Chest Compressions**

This lesson teaches you how to perform chest compressions while the neonate is receiving positive-pressure ventilation. You must have demonstrated competence in bag-and-mask ventilation prior to beginning this lesson.

Lesson 5   **Endotracheal Intubation**

This lesson teaches the knowledge and skills necessary to assist with and perform an intubation of a neonate. The first part describes the sequence of activities. The second part, a study guide, provides specific directions for step-by-step practice of the skills involved, using an infant intubation manikin.

Lesson 6   **Medications**

This lesson presents information on the drugs and volume expanders that may be used when resuscitating a neonate. The recommended concentration and preparation of each medication is discussed as well as what drugs to use in specific circumstances and the correct dosage and route of each.

Objectives and Testing

Each lesson contains objectives related to the specific part of the resuscitation procedure presented in that lesson. These objectives generally are one of two types:

Knowledge

Information (or Knowledge) Objectives

These objectives have to do with recalling and using the information given in the lesson. Your knowledge will be tested in the practice activities and posttest in each lesson.

Performance

Clinical Performance Objectives

These objectives have to do with the ability to perform a given procedure at an acceptable level of skill. Your skill will be tested through the use of performance checklists found at the end of certain lessons.

Completion of each lesson depends on successfully passing the written posttest and, if the lesson contains one, the performance checklist.

The following table lists the evaluation process for each part of the program.

Testing of Each Lesson Includes the Following:

Lessons	Written Posttest	Performance Evaluation
Lesson 1 — Introduction to the Program	X	
Lesson 2 — Initial Steps in Resuscitation	X	X
Lesson 3A — Bag and Mask: Equipment	X	
Lesson 3B — Bag and Mask: Ventilation	X	X
Lesson 3C — Bag and Mask: Procedure	X	X
Lesson 4 — Chest Compressions	X	X
Lesson 5 — Endotracheal Intubation	X	X
Lesson 6 — Medications	X	

Level of Responsibility

Although we have listed all the lessons in the program, you will need to work through only the ones that are appropriate to *your* level of responsibility. Resuscitation responsibilities vary from hospital to hospital, and within an institution are different for various members of the resuscitation team. In some hospitals, nurses may have the responsibility of intubating an infant, but in other hospitals, physicians or respiratory therapists may do this. How far you need to go in this program will depend upon your role in the institution where you work.

Prior to beginning the program, you must have a very clear idea of your exact responsibilities. If you have any questions as to the level of your responsibilities in a resuscitation, see your instructor or charge nurse before beginning the program.

Neonatal resuscitation is most effective when performed by a designated team. It is important for you to know the neonatal resuscitation responsibilities of team members who are working with you. Be sure that you are clear about what to expect of them as you work together to resuscitate an infant.

Note:

This program introduces the concepts and basic skills of neonatal resuscitation. Completion of the program does not imply that an individual has acquired the necessary competence to perform neonatal resuscitation. Supervised clinical experience is required for an individual to assume responsibility for any portion of neonatal resuscitation. Each hospital is responsible for determining the level of competence and qualifications required for an individual to assume clinical responsibility for neonatal resuscitation.

The content of this program conforms to the published guidelines for neonatal resuscitation *(JAMA* 1986;255:2969–2973). The flowchart sequences were developed from these guidelines and instructional experience. The guidelines represent a consensus of experienced physicians, nurses, and other scientists. The guidelines are largely based on scientific data; where data are scant, the guidelines represent the best current opinion of experienced individuals.

This program can be an entry level course. Completion of a course in Basic Life Support (BLS) is not required but may be desirable.

Universal Precautions

The US Centers for Disease Control have recommended that universal precautions be taken whenever risk of exposure to blood or bodily fluids is high and the potential infectious status of the patient is unknown, as is certainly the case in neonatal resuscitation.

All fluid products from patients (i.e., blood, urine, stool, saliva, vomitus, etc.) should be treated as potentially infectious. Therefore, gloves should be worn when resuscitating a newborn infant, and personnel should not use their mouth to apply suction via a DeLee or any other suction device. Mouth-to-mouth resuscitation should not be performed, and a bag-mask device should always be available for use during resuscitation. Masks and protective eye wear or face shields should be worn during procedures that are likely to generate droplets of blood or other bodily fluids. Gowns and aprons should be worn during procedures that will probably generate splashes of blood or other bodily fluids. It is essential that delivery rooms be equipped with resuscitation bags, masks, laryngoscopes, endotracheal tubes, mechanical suction devices, and the necessary protective shields.

Overview of Resuscitation in the Delivery Room

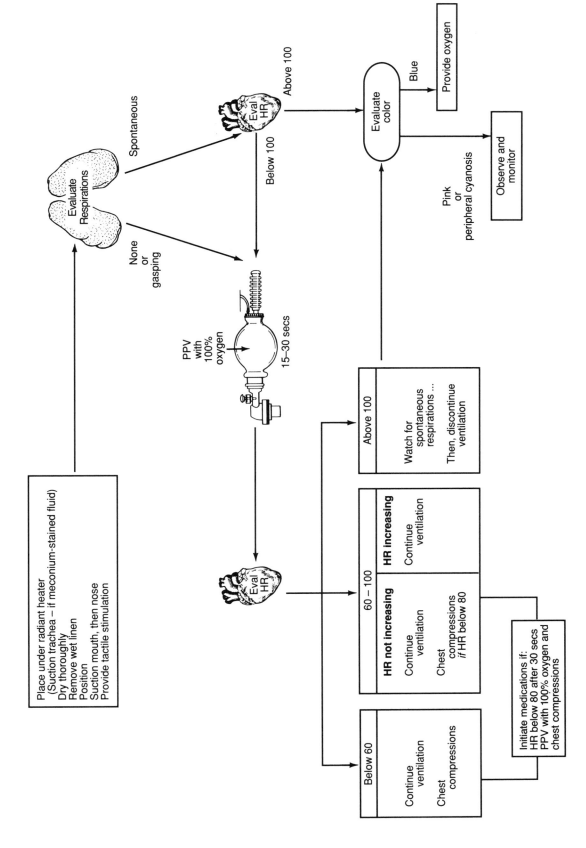

Introduction to the Program

Contents

Introduction to the Program

Lesson 1

Overview of Lesson 1

This lesson, which is the first in the program, contains important information on a series of topics related to resuscitating newborns. Some basic concepts of the physiology of asphyxia are presented first. Later sections describe how you might identify, prior to delivery, the infant who may need resuscitation at birth. You will learn what preparations should be made in the delivery room for both an expected "normal" infant and one at risk for asphyxia. Other topics presented include: the signs used to evaluate an infant at birth and throughout a resuscitative effort; the proper sequence of the procedure, following the time-honored ABCs of resuscitation; and the elements that contribute to a successful resuscitation.

Objectives

When you have completed Lesson 1, you will be able to:
- Identify the major characteristics of primary and secondary apnea.
- Briefly describe why apnea at birth must be regarded as secondary apnea.
- Identify correct statements and definitions regarding pulmonary perfusion and asphyxia.
- Identify correct concepts in anticipating and being prepared for resuscitation in the delivery room.
- List the three primary signs used for evaluating an infant during resuscitation.
- Identify the appropriate and inappropriate use of the Apgar score in resuscitating a newborn at birth.
- List the ABCs of resuscitation and identify which actions in a resuscitation relate to which of the ABCs.

These objectives are all "knowledge" objectives, which will be tested using the posttest at the end of the lesson.

Decision Table

If ...	Then ...
You feel you can pass a test on these objectives ...	Turn to the posttest on page 1-32.
You wish to know more before attempting the test ...	Go on to the next page.

Physiology of Asphyxia — Apnea

Before we go into the details of teaching the resuscitation process, let's take a look at several concepts basic to the physiology of asphyxia. An understanding of this physiology will help you select an appropriate approach to resuscitating an individual infant.

First, we will consider the physiologic changes that occur with mild and severe asphyxia. You will also learn that these changes may occur in the fetus as well as in the newly born infant.

The next section presents the normal physiologic changes that occur in the lungs at delivery and describes how such changes may be affected by asphyxia.

Apnea

When infants become asphyxiated (either in utero or following delivery), they undergo a well-defined sequence of events.

Primary Apnea

When a fetus or infant is deprived of oxygen, an initial period of rapid breathing occurs. If the asphyxia continues, the respiratory movements cease, the heart rate begins to fall, and the infant enters a period of apnea known as *primary* apnea. Exposure to oxygen and stimulation during the period of primary apnea in most instances will induce respirations.

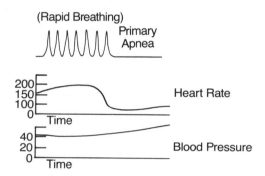

Secondary Apnea

If the asphyxia continues, the infant develops deep gasping respirations, the heart rate continues to decrease, and the blood pressure begins to fall. The respirations become weaker and weaker until the infant takes a last gasp and enters a period of apnea called *secondary* apnea. During secondary apnea the heart rate, blood pressure, and oxygen in the blood (Pao_2) continue to fall farther and farther. The infant now is unresponsive to stimulation, and artificial ventilation with oxygen (positive-pressure ventilation) must be initiated at once.

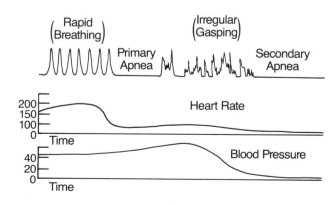

It is very important to realize that once the child is in secondary apnea, the longer you delay starting ventilation, the longer it will take the infant to develop spontaneous respirations. Even a very short delay in initiating artificial ventilation can result in a very long delay in establishing spontaneous and regular respirations. Also, and of great importance, the longer an infant is in secondary apnea, the greater is the chance that brain damage will occur.

Primary vs. Secondary Apnea

It is important to note that, as a result of fetal hypoxia, the infant may go through primary apnea and into secondary apnea while in utero. Thus an infant may be born in either primary or secondary apnea. In a clinical setting, primary and secondary apnea are virtually indistinguishable from one another. In both instances the infant is not breathing, and the heart rate may be below 100 per minute.

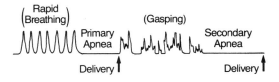

The fetus may go through primary and into secondary apnea while in utero. *Thus when an infant is apneic at birth, one cannot easily tell whether the baby is in primary or secondary apnea.*

A newborn infant in *primary* apnea will reestablish a breathing pattern (although irregular and possibly ineffective) without intervention. An infant in *secondary* apnea will not resume breathing of his or her own accord. Positive-pressure ventilation will be required to establish respirations.

If we could identify which infants are in primary apnea and which are in secondary apnea, it would be easy to differentiate those infants needing simple stimulation and exposure to oxygen from those requiring positive-pressure ventilation. However, we cannot easily clinically distinguish primary from secondary apnea at birth.

Assume Secondary Apnea

This means that *when we are faced with an apneic infant at delivery, we must assume that we are dealing with secondary apnea, and resuscitation should begin immediately.* To assume, incorrectly, that an infant has primary apnea and to provide stimulation that is ineffective will only lead to delayed oxygenation and increased risk of brain damage.

Physiology of Asphyxia — The Lungs and the Circulation

During intrauterine life, the lungs serve no ventilatory purpose because the placenta supplies the fetus with oxygen. At the time of birth, however, several changes need to take place for the lungs to take over the vital function of supplying the body with oxygen. Here we will discuss the changes that must occur for normal respiration to be established and how these changes are compromised in some infants. This information will provide you with a greater understanding of the need for prompt and appropriate intervention in the asphyxiated infant.

Fetus

Since the oxygen supplied to the fetus comes from the placenta, the lungs contain no air. The alveoli (air sacs) of the fetus are filled instead with fluid that has been produced by the lungs.

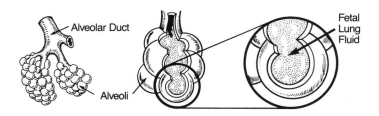

Since fetal lungs are fluid filled and do not contain oxygen, blood passing through the lungs cannot pick up oxygen to deliver throughout the body. Thus, blood flow through the lungs is markedly diminished compared to that which is required following birth. Diminished blood flow through the lungs of the fetus is a result of the partial closing of the arterioles in the lungs. This results in the majority of blood flow being diverted away from the lungs through the ductus arteriosus.

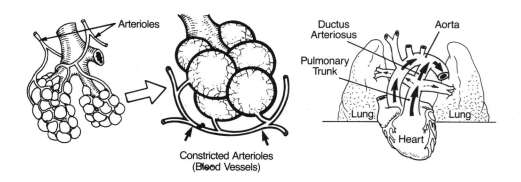

Diminished Blood Flow Through Fetal Lungs

Birth

At birth, as the infant takes the first few breaths, several changes occur whereby the lungs take over the lifelong function of supplying the body with oxygen.

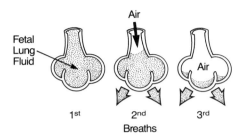

Following birth, the lungs expand as they are filled with air. The fetal lung fluid gradually leaves the alveoli.

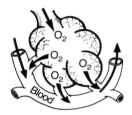

Arterioles Dilate and Blood Flow Increases

At the same time as the lungs are expanding and the fetal lung fluid is clearing, the arterioles in the lungs begin to open, allowing a considerable increase in the amount of blood flowing through the lungs.

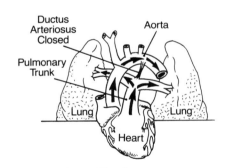

Pulmonary Blood Flow Increases

Blood previously diverted through the ductus arteriosus flows through the lungs where it picks up oxygen to transport to tissues throughout the body. Soon there is no need for the ductus, and it eventually closes.

In an attempt to establish normal respirations, the infant can develop problems in two areas:
- Fluid may remain in the alveoli;
- Blood flow to the lungs may not increase as desired.
Let's look at each of these problems individually.

Fetal Lung Fluid

At birth, the alveoli are filled with "fetal lung fluid." It takes a considerable amount of pressure in the lungs to overcome the fluid forces and open the alveoli for the first time. In fact, the first several breaths may require *two to three* times the pressure required for succeeding breaths.

Approximately one-third of fetal lung fluid is removed during vaginal delivery as the chest is squeezed and lung fluid exits through the nose and mouth. The remaining fluid passes through the alveoli into the lymphatics surrounding the lungs. How quickly fluid leaves the lungs depends on the *effectiveness* of the first few breaths.

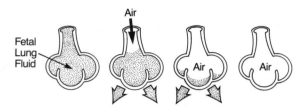

Fortunately, the first few breaths of most newborn infants are generally effective, expanding the alveoli and replacing the lung fluid with air.

Problems Clearing Fluid

Problems in clearing lung fluid occur in infants whose lungs do not inflate well with the first few breaths. These are:
• Apnea at birth
• Weak initial respiratory effort

Apnea at Birth

With an infant who has never taken an initial breath, you can assume that no expansion of alveoli has occurred and the lungs remain filled with fluid. When providing artificial ventilation to such an infant, additional pressure is often required to begin the process of expanding alveoli and clearing lung fluid.

Weak Respiratory Effort

Shallow, ineffective respirations may occur in premature infants or in infants who are depressed as a result of asphyxia, maternal drugs, or anesthesia. The gasping, irregular respirations that follow primary apnea may not be sufficient to properly expand the lungs. This means that you cannot rely on the presence of spontaneous respirations as an indicator of effective respiration in the newborn.

Pulmonary Circulation

It is not enough, however, merely to have air entering the lungs. There must be an adequate supply of blood flowing through the capillaries of the lungs so that oxygen can pass into the blood and be carried throughout the body. This requires a considerable increase in the amount of blood flowing through (perfusing) the lungs at birth.

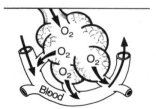

**Normal Pulmonary Perfusion
(Blood Flow)**

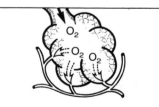

**Decreased Pulmonary Perfusion
(Blood Flow)**

Decreased Pulmonary Perfusion

Asphyxia results in a low oxygen content of the blood (hypoxemia) with a resulting fall in pH (acidosis). In the presence of hypoxemia and acidosis, the arterioles of the newborn's lungs remain constricted, and the ductus remains open. Fetal circulation is maintained with no increase in pulmonary blood flow. Blood that should be perfusing the lungs continues to flow through the ductus.

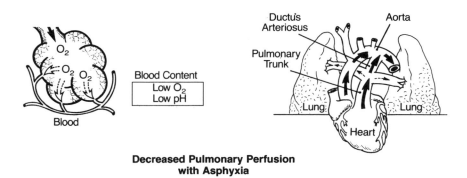

**Decreased Pulmonary Perfusion
with Asphyxia**

As long as decreased pulmonary perfusion exists, proper oxygenation of the tissues of the body is impossible — even when the infant is being properly ventilated. **Remember, oxygenation depends not only on oxygen reaching the alveoli but also on pulmonary blood flow (perfusion).**

Mild Asphyxia

In *mildly* asphyxiated infants whose O_2 and pH are only slightly lowered, it may be possible to increase pulmonary perfusion by acting quickly and properly ventilating the infant with 100% oxygen.

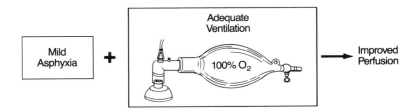

Severe Asphyxia

Pulmonary perfusion in *severely* asphyxiated infants with severe metabolic acidosis may not improve with ventilation alone. The combination of ventilation and administration of sodium bicarbonate to increase pH may result in opening of the pulmonary arterioles and thus improvement in pulmonary perfusion. However, the role of sodium bicarbonate and other medications in the management of poor pulmonary perfusion is not yet clear.

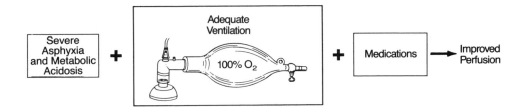

Severe asphyxia may be present at birth, or it may occur as a result of delayed or improperly administered resuscitative efforts.

Pulmonary Vasoconstriction

A term commonly used to refer to decreased pulmonary blood flow in the asphyxiated infant is **pulmonary vasoconstriction.**

Pulmonary **(Of the Lungs)**	+	**Vaso-** **(Vascular or Vessels)**	+	**Constriction** **(Constricted)**

This refers to the constriction of the vessels of the lungs. The vessels that open in the lungs of a normal infant remain in a constricted state in an asphyxiated infant.

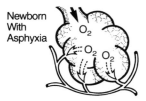
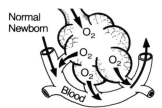

Newborn With Asphyxia

Vessel — Constricted
Blood Flow — Decreased

Normal Newborn

Vessel — Open
Blood Flow — Increased

Cardiac Function and Circulation

Early in asphyxia, arterioles in the bowels, kidneys, muscles, and skin constrict. The resulting redistribution of blood flow helps preserve function by preferentially supplying oxygen and substrates to the heart and brain.

As asphyxia is prolonged, there is deterioration of myocardial function and cardiac output. Blood flow to vital organs is reduced. This sets the stage for progressive organ damage.

Summary

Below is a summary of the important concepts presented on the physiology of asphyxia.

Primary Apnea

Infants who become asphyxiated either in utero or following birth undergo a definite sequence of events. There is an initial period of rapid gasping, then respirations cease, heart rate begins to fall, and *primary* apnea follows. If the asphyxia continues, there are deep gasping respirations, the heart rate continues to fall, and blood pressure begins to fall.

Secondary Apnea

The gasping respirations become weaker and weaker until the infant takes a last gasp and enters *secondary* apnea. The heart rate and arterial pressure continue to fall, and positive-pressure ventilation must be given.
With secondary apnea, the longer the delay in starting ventilation:
• The longer it will take to establish spontaneous respirations;
• The greater will be the chance of brain damage.

Assume Secondary Apnea

Primary and secondary apnea are virtually indistinguishable from one another. Therefore, apnea at birth should be treated as secondary apnea, and resuscitation should be initiated immediately. The entire sequence with regard to primary and secondary apnea may begin in utero and continue after delivery.

Clearing Fetal Lung Fluid

Fetal lung fluid must be cleared if air is to fill the lungs. To clear fetal lung fluid and expand the lungs requires *two to three* times the pressure of a normal breath.

Problems in clearing lung fluid occur in:

- Infants apneic at birth;
- Infants with weak initial respiratory effort:
  - Premature infants,
  - Infants depressed by asphyxia, maternal drugs, or anesthesia.

Chest movement cannot be used as the *sole* indicator of effective respiration.

Pulmonary Circulation

At birth, pulmonary blood flow must increase for proper oxygenation. This is accomplished by arterioles in the lungs opening and filling with blood previously diverted away from the lungs through the ductus arteriosus.

Decreased Pulmonary Perfusion

In the asphyxiated newborn, hypoxemia and acidosis maintain a fetal pattern of circulation with diminished pulmonary blood flow.

Cardiac Function and Circulation

Early in asphyxia, blood is shunted to the brain and the heart. With increasing hypoxemia and acidosis, myocardial function fails, cardiac output decreases, and blood flow even to these vital organs is diminished.

Practice Activity 1

The practice activities in each of the lessons of this program are included so that you will have a means of evaluating your progress toward the stated objectives. These practice activities also will focus attention on the key concepts and principles and will thus help you review the material you have read. Follow the directions given for various parts of the practice activities and complete each item.

Fill In

Complete each item by filling in the appropriate word or words.

1. Why should all apnea at birth be treated as secondary apnea?

_____

_____

_____

Matching

Match the types of apnea with the descriptive statements in the first column. Some of the statements apply to *both* types, so you will use both **A** and **B** for these statements.

2. _____ Infant is not breathing   **A.** Primary apnea

3. _____ Blood pressure falls profoundly   **B.** Secondary apnea

4. _____ Infant will not resume breathing on his or her own

5. _____ Heart rate falls

6. _____ Infant will resume breathing on his or her own

7. _____ Can occur in utero

True/False

Use a **T** or **F** to show whether each statement is **true** or **false.**

8. _____ During secondary apnea, exposure to oxygen and stimulation usually will bring about respirations.

9. _____ An infant subjected to fetal hypoxemia may go through primary apnea and into secondary apnea while in utero.

10. _____ Once a child is in secondary apnea, even a very short delay in starting ventilation can result in a very long delay in establishing spontaneous and regular respirations.

11. _____ When an infant is apneic at birth, it usually is easy to tell whether the baby is in primary or secondary apnea.

12. _____ In all infants, fetal lung fluid is cleared from the alveoli following the first few breaths.

13. _____ It takes a considerable amount of pressure to expand the lungs and clear the fetal lung fluid.

14. _____ The first few breaths after birth require five to six times the intrathoracic pressure of a normal breath.

15. _____ With progressive asphyxia, myocardial function fails and cardiac output falls.

16. _____ If you deliver adequate amounts of oxygen to an infant's lungs, this is all that is really necessary for proper oxygenation.

17. _____ The hypoxemia and acidosis resulting from asphyxia can lead to pulmonary vasoconstriction and decreased pulmonary blood flow.

18. _____ Pulmonary blood flow must increase following delivery in order for proper oxygenation to occur.

Matching

Match the terms in the right-hand column with the correct definitions in the left-hand column. (You will not use all of the terms.)

Definitions

19. _____ A narrowing or contraction of the blood vessels of the lungs

20. _____ A decreased flow of blood through the capillaries of the lungs

21. _____ The flow of blood through the capillaries of the lungs

22. _____ A lack of oxygen

Terms

A. Asphyxia

B. Decreased pulmonary perfusion

C. Intrathoracic pressure

D. Pulmonary perfusion

E. Pulmonary vasoconstriction

F. Respiratory effort

Practice Activity 1: Answers

The correct answers to the items in the practice activity are provided so that you can check the accuracy of your own responses. With each practice activity in this program, after you have checked the answers, *review thoroughly* the material that covers any questions you missed or about which you had some question. It is important that you master the information given in each section of the lesson before you proceed.

Fill In

1. At the outset, you cannot tell the difference between these two types of apnea.

   The consequences and complications of untreated secondary apnea are severe (brain damage, death); therefore, one cannot assume that the apnea present is primary. If apnea is observed, it must be treated as secondary apnea.

Matching

2. A, B

3. B

4. B

5. A, B

6. A

7. A, B

True/False

8. **False** — This is true of *primary* apnea. An infant in *secondary* apnea is unresponsive to stimulation.

9. **True**

10. **True**

11. **False** — Primary and secondary apnea are very difficult to distinguish from one another in a clinical situation.

12. **False** — The rate in which fetal lung fluid is cleared from the alveoli varies, depending on the forcefulness of the first few breaths.

13. **True**

14. **False** — The actual amount is closer to two to three times the pressure of a normal breath — which is still a considerable amount.

15. **True**

16. **False** — Oxygen to the lungs is not enough. There must be adequate ventilation and a continuous flow of blood through the capillaries of the lungs to assure that sufficient amounts of oxygen will be circulated to tissues throughout the body.

17. **True**

18. **True**

Matching

19. E

20. B

21. D

22. A

Decision

If . . .	Then . . .
You missed no more than 2 questions . . .	Congratulations! You have demonstrated good knowledge of the key concepts of the physiology of asphyxia. Clear up any questions you may have, then go on to the next section.
You missed 3 or more answers . . .	Study carefully the information for the questions you missed. Try again to answer those questions; then go ahead to the next section. If you have any further questions, see your instructor or supervisor.

Being Prepared for Resuscitation

We have discussed the importance of intervening quickly when a newborn infant is in need of resuscitation.

In order for prompt, effective intervention to take place, two major factors must be given proper attention. These two factors are:

- Anticipating the need for resuscitation;
- Adequate preparation, both of equipment and personnel.

Let's look at each of these two factors.

Anticipation

Asphyxiation in a newborn at birth may come as a surprise. However, most newborn asphyxia can be anticipated. When unanticipated, resuscitation can be promptly and effectively initiated only if the proper equipment is readily available and a well-trained team is on hand.

This does not mean that asphyxia in a neonate will occur every time it is anticipated. Some infants, in spite of being at risk for asphyxia, will do well following delivery and will require no resuscitative assistance. If, however, every time asphyxia is anticipated the infant actually requires resuscitation, then it is clear that the cases are not being screened thoroughly. The delivery room staff should be prepared to handle *more* problems than they actually encounter.

Antepartum/ Intrapartum History

Delivery of a depressed or asphyxiated infant can be anticipated in many cases on the basis of information found in both the antepartum and the intrapartum histories.

Antepartum Factors

Maternal diabetes
Pregnancy-induced hypertension
Chronic hypertension
Previous Rh sensitization
Previous stillbirth
Bleeding in second or third trimester
Maternal infection
Hydramnios
Oligohydramnios

Post-term gestation
Multiple gestation
Size–dates discrepancy
Drug therapy, e.g.:
   Reserpine
   Lithium carbonate
   Magnesium
   Adrenergic — blocking drugs
Maternal drug abuse

Intrapartum Factors

Elective or emergency cesarean section
Abnormal presentation
Premature labor
Rupture of membranes more than
   24 hours prior to delivery
Foul-smelling amniotic fluid
Precipitous labor
Prolonged labor (greater than 24 hours)
Prolonged second stage of labor
   (greater than 2 hours)

Non-reassuring fetal heart rate
   patterns
Use of general anesthesia
Uterine tetany
Narcotics administered to
   mother within 4 hours of
   delivery
Meconium-stained amniotic fluid
Prolapsed cord
Abruptio placenta
Placenta previa

It should be obvious that some of these factors may present during a delivery. Thus, you must have the factors well in mind so that if they occur, you will recognize that asphyxia is a potential problem.

Adequate Preparation

In spite of the screening of cases through review of the antepartum and intrapartum histories, there will be occasions when the birth of an asphyxiated infant has not been anticipated. To allow for such situations, the minimum preparation for any delivery should include:

- A radiant warmer, heated and ready for use,
- All resuscitation equipment *immediately* available and in working order,
- At least one person skilled in neonatal resuscitation should be present in the delivery room; one or two other persons should be available to assist with an emergency resuscitation.

Equipment

All of the equipment necessary for a complete resuscitation must be present in the delivery room and be fully operational. In cases of an anticipated asphyxiated infant, all of the equipment should also be removed from its packages and ready to use. If there is concern about the cost involved in opening packages of sterile equipment that may not be used, keep this in mind: it is far less expensive to resterilize an unused bag and mask or endotracheal tube than to deal with the long-term financial, emotional, and social consequences of an infant damaged as the result of a delay in initiating appropriate therapy.

In the event of a multiple gestation, a full complement of equipment, as well as staff, must be available for *each* anticipated infant.

A complete list of neonatal resuscitation equipment is included in the appendix at the end of this lesson.

Personnel

For "Normal" Deliveries

At *every* delivery, there should be at least one person (physician, nurse, respiratory therapist, etc.) who has the skills required to perform a complete resuscitation. He or she must be skilled in ventilation with bag and mask, endotracheal intubation, chest compressions, and the use of medications. Often this person is the one delivering the infant, but it may be someone else.

When the individual with skills to perform a complete resuscitation is caring for the mother, another person who is capable of initiating and assisting with a resuscitation must be present in the delivery room and must be primarily responsible for the infant. This latter individual must be present even in cases in which a normal, *healthy* infant is expected.

Let's see how these two people might work together in a situation where resuscitation is needed. A delivery room nurse present is skilled in suctioning, tactile stimulation of an infant, providing bag-and-mask ventilation, and performing chest compressions. This nurse might initially suction the infant, provide tactile stimulation, and evaluate the respirations and heart rate. If the infant does not respond appropriately, bag-and-mask ventilation and, if necessary, chest compressions may be initiated by the nurse. The other person would assist with ventilation and chest compressions and also would, if the situation warranted, take the additional steps of endotracheal intubation and administration of medications.

It is not sufficient to have someone "on call" (either at the individual's home or a remote area of the hospital) for infant resuscitations in the delivery room. When resuscitation is needed, it must be initiated *without delay;* there is absolutely no time to wait for someone to be called when an infant needs resuscitation.

When Asphyxia Is Anticipated

We have been discussing preparations that should be made in anticipation of a healthy infant. When neonatal asphyxia is likely, two individuals capable of working together as a team to perform all aspects of a resuscitation should be present in the delivery room. The only responsibility of these two people should be that of managing the infant. This means that the individual managing the mother is not to be regarded as one of the two. These two people might include a respiratory therapist and a nurse, or nurse and pediatrician, or two nurses. Whatever the combination, one of the two must be skilled in endotracheal intubation and administration of medications.

Remember, with multiple births, such a team is needed for each infant.

Summary

Two major factors for prompt, effective resuscitation are:
- Anticipation of need for resuscitation,
- Adequate preparation of equipment and personnel.

Anticipation

Most neonatal resuscitations can be anticipated.
- Delivery room staff should be prepared to handle problems more often than they are actually encountered.
- Delivery of asphyxiated infants often can be anticipated on the basis of the antepartum and intrapartum histories.

Preparation

To allow for the occasional unexpected case of an infant who is asphyxiated, the *minimum* preparation for *every* delivery should include:
- A radiant warmer, heated and ready for use;
- All resuscitation equipment *immediately* available and in working order;
- At least one person skilled in neonatal resuscitation in the delivery room; one or two other persons should be available to assist with an emergency resuscitation.

When an asphyxiated infant is anticipated, two individuals capable of working together as a team to perform all aspects of a resuscitation should be present in the delivery room. The only responsibility of these two individuals should be to manage the infant.

Practice Activity 2

As before, respond to each item in the practice activity, following the directions given.

True/False

1. _____ Many problems of asphyxiation at the time of birth can be anticipated.

2. _____ Delivery of an asphyxiated infant can always be anticipated by a thorough review of the antepartum and intrapartum histories.

3. _____ A *full* set of resuscitation equipment should be present in the delivery room only when the need for resuscitation is anticipated.

4. _____ There should be present at *every* delivery at least one person capable of performing a complete resuscitation (including intubation and administration of medications).

5. _____ It is sufficient to have someone "on call" within the hospital to perform such procedures as endotracheal intubation and administration of medications.

6. _____ If an asphyxiated infant is anticipated, two people capable of working together as a team to perform all aspects of a resuscitation should be present at the delivery, and their *only* responsibility should be that of managing the infant.

Practice Activity 2: Answers

Compare your responses to the ones given below.

True/False

1. True

2. False—Neonatal asphyxia cannot be anticipated in all cases, even with careful review of the maternal record.

3. False—The equipment should be in the delivery room and ready for use in *every* delivery.

4. True

5. False—When resuscitation is needed, it must be initiated without delay. There is no time to wait for someone to be called when an infant is in need of resuscitation.

6. True

Decision

If . . .	Then . . .
You had at least 5 correct answers . . .	Good! Go right on to the next section.
You missed 2 or more of the answers . . .	Review as needed, then try again to answer the questions you missed. If you need help, contact your instructor or supervisor.

The Action/Evaluation/Decision Cycle

A very important aspect of resuscitation is evaluating the infant, deciding what action to take, and then taking action. Further evaluation data is the basis for more decisions and further actions. This cycle can be represented by the following diagram.

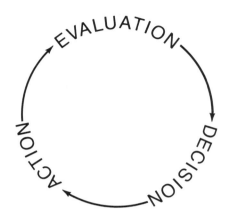

The Cycle

Efficient and effective resuscitation is brought about through a series of actions, evaluations, decisions, and further actions. As an example, at one point while you are providing tactile stimulation, you will evaluate the infant's respirations. On the basis of that evaluation, you will decide what action to take next.

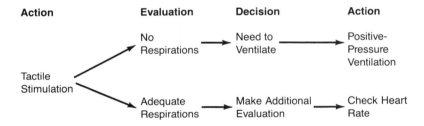

If your evaluation of the respirations indicates that the infant is not breathing or that the respirations are inadequate, you have the basis for deciding that the next action is to provide positive-pressure ventilation. If, on the other hand, the respirations are normal, the next action should be to evaluate the infant's heart rate.

After the initiation of any action, you must evaluate its effect on the neonate and make a decision about the next step.

Signs to Evaluate

The Apgar score is not used in determining when to initiate a resuscitation or in making decisions regarding the course of a resuscitation. Evaluation is primarily based on the following three signs:

- Respirations
- Heart rate
- Color

Apgar Score

The Apgar score is an objective method of evaluating the newborn's condition. It is generally performed at 1 minute and again at 5 minutes of age. However, assessment of the infant should begin immediately at birth. If the infant requires interventions based on assessment of respirations, heart rate, or color, they should be instituted promptly. Such interventions should not be delayed until an Apgar score is assigned at 1 minute. A delay could be of critical importance, particularly in the severely asphyxiated infant.

While the Apgar score is not useful as a basis for decision-making at the beginning of resuscitation, it may be helpful for assessing the infant's condition and the effectiveness of the resuscitative effort. Thus, an Apgar score should be assigned at 1 and 5 minutes of age. When the 5-minute Apgar score is less than 7, additional scores should be obtained every 5 minutes for up to 20 minutes or until two successive scores are 8 or greater.

The ABCs of Resuscitation

The steps in resuscitating newborn infants follow the well-known "ABCs" of resuscitation.

A—Establish an open *airway*

B—Initiate *breathing*

C—Maintain *circulation*

The components of the neonatal resuscitation procedure as related to the ABCs of resuscitation are shown here.

A—Establish an open *airway:*

• Position the infant.

• Suction the mouth, nose, and in some instances, the trachea.

• If necessary, insert an endotracheal tube to assure an open airway.

B—Initiate *breathing:*

• Use tactile stimulation to initiate respirations.

• Employ positive-pressure ventilation when necessary, using either:
  • Bag and mask, or
  • Bag and endotracheal tube.

C—Maintain *circulation:*

• Stimulate and maintain the circulation of blood with:
  • Chest compressions, and
  • Medications.

Organization

Rather than teaching the resuscitation procedure all at once, we are going to divide the procedure into its major parts and teach each part individually. This will allow you to focus on each phase. Also, this organization allows you to use only the lessons that deal with the knowledge and skills needed to carry out your specific level of responsibility.

Practice Activity 3

Work through each item carefully as you evaluate your knowledge of key ideas in the previous two sections.

Fill In

List the ABCs of resuscitation.

1. **A:** _____

2. **B:** _____

3. **C:** _____

The basic components of the neonatal resuscitation procedure are listed below. For each component, indicate which of the ABCs of resuscitation it helps bring about. (Enter **A, B,** or **C** in the blank.)

4. _____ Use of bag and mask

5. _____ Medications

6. _____ Insertion of an endotracheal tube

7. _____ Positioning the infant

8. _____ Tactile stimulation

9. _____ Chest compressions

10. _____ Suctioning the infant

11. _____ Positive-pressure ventilation

12–14. Resuscitative decisions are primarily based on what three signs?

• _____

• _____

• _____

True/False

15. _____ Because the Apgar score is not assigned until 1 minute after birth, it is not useful as a basis for making decisions about the initiation of resuscitation.

16. _____ There is no need to obtain Apgar scores in infants who require resuscitation.

Practice Activity 3: Answers

Check your answers carefully, then review as needed.

Fill In

1. **A:** Establish an open *airway*

2. **B:** Initiate *breathing*

3. **C:** Maintain *circulation*

4. **B**

5. **C**

6. **A**

7. **A**

8. **B**

9. **C**

10. **A**

11. **B**

12–14. • Respirations
• Heart rate
• Color

True/False

15. **True**

16. **False** — Although not used to initiate resuscitation, Apgar scores help indicate the infant's condition and how effective the resuscitative efforts have been

Decision

If . . .	Then . . .
Your score was 15 or more . . .	You are doing well. Proceed to the next section on principles of a successful resuscitation.
You missed more than 2 . . .	Review the information having to do with the questions you missed, then take the test again.

Principles of a Successful Resuscitation

A successful resuscitation depends on anticipating or immediately recognizing the infant in need of resuscitation, initiating the procedure promptly, and performing procedures skillfully. The consequences that occur when a resuscitation is not handled well are outlined here, along with the principles that lead to resuscitating an infant in an efficient and effective manner.

Consequences

Delayed or ineffective resuscitative efforts can:
- Make the resuscitation more difficult.
- Increase the likelihood of brain damage,

Difficult Resuscitation

The longer an infant is allowed to go without adequate resuscitation, the more difficult the resuscitation becomes.

When resuscitation is delayed or incorrectly performed, resuscitating the infant will take longer and be harder than if prompt, appropriate action had been taken. Quickly clearing the airway and skillfully providing a brief period of ventilation may maintain oxygenation and pulmonary perfusion, thereby negating the need for chest compressions and/or medications.

Brain Damage

An insufficient amount of oxygen can result in brain damage.

The brain must have a constant supply of oxygen in order to function properly. The longer the brain remains without oxygen, the greater the chance that irreparable damage to cells will occur.

Damage to other organs also can result from inadequate oxygen. In addition to the brain, those organs most likely to suffer damage are the bowel, lungs, kidneys, and heart.

Principles of Success

The following five principles, if followed closely, will increase the likelihood of a successful resuscitation.

Readily Available Personnel/Team

Personnel adequately trained in neonatal resuscitation should be physically present at every delivery.

This should be the case even when a normal birth of a healthy infant is anticipated. One can never be certain that the need for resuscitation won't arise. *It is not necessary for everyone in the delivery room to be capable of performing all aspects of a complete resuscitation.* But each person should know what his or her specific responsibilities are, and he or she must be capable of carrying them out.

Skilled Practitioners

Personnel in the delivery room must not only know what they have to do, but they must be able to do it efficiently and effectively.

The required skills must be practiced *before* they are to be used in the delivery room. Also, steps should be taken to be certain that the skills (and the related knowledge) are maintained through frequent use or scheduled practice.

Coordinated Team

Personnel involved in resuscitating an infant must work together as a coordinated team or unit.

This concept is important throughout all stages of the resuscitative effort. Personnel must not only possess the skills and know exactly what their responsibilities are, but they must be able to coordinate their efforts for an efficient and effective resuscitation.

Resuscitation Tailored to Patient Response

The initial resuscitation procedures should be initiated promptly, and each further step must be selected on the basis of specific patient response.

Neonatal resuscitation is *not* one procedure applicable to all infants, nor is it a collection of random events. The total resuscitation procedure is made up of a unified and coordinated series of steps. Each succeeding step logically follows the previous one, based on an evaluation of the infant's condition and response.

Available and Functioning Equipment

Wherever newborn infants are cared for in a hospital, appropriate resuscitation equipment should be immediately available and in working order.

The consequences resulting from a delay in initiating therapy can be devastating. The cost of having appropriate resuscitation equipment and drugs at hand cannot begin to match the cost of a damaged infant.

Practice Activity 4

Use this practice activity to test your knowledge of the key concepts and principles of a successful resuscitation.

Fill In

State the two major consequences of delayed or ineffective resuscitative efforts.

1–2. • _____

_____

• _____

_____

True/False

3. _____ The individuals resuscitating an infant must be able to coordinate their efforts as a team.

4. _____ Delivery room personnel must acquire, practice, and maintain the skills necessary for efficient and effective resuscitation.

5. _____ Wherever newborn infants are cared for in a hospital, appropriate and functional equipment should be immediately available.

6. _____ Neonatal resuscitation is a procedure in which the same actions are carried out regardless of the response of the infant.

7. _____ An infant can do without oxygen for a considerable length of time before there is any danger of brain damage.

8. _____ A lack of oxygen can damage the kidneys, lungs, heart, and bowel.

Practice Activity 4: Answers

Compare your answers to the ones given below, then review as necessary.

Fill In

1–2. • Increased chance of brain damage

• Increased difficulty of the resuscitation

True/False

3. True

4. True

5. True

6. False — The flow of a resuscitation is based on the response of the infant to any particular action. This will change from infant to infant.

7. False — If the brain is deprived of oxygen for even a very short time, irreparable damage can result.

8. True

Decision

If . . .	Then . . .
You were able to answer at least 7 of the items correctly . . .	Very good! You may want to take time to review the key points in this introductory lesson before you take the posttest.
You had 2 or more of the items incorrect . . .	You should review the material that covers the questions you missed. Then try again to answer those questions. Take time to review the main ideas in the lesson before you go on to the posttest.

Posttest
Lesson 1—Introduction to the Program

Name _____ Date _____

This posttest will help you identify your understanding of the information presented in Lesson 1.

Matching

Match the types of apnea with the descriptive statements in the first column. Some of the statements apply to *both* types, so you will use both "A" and "B" for these statements.

1. _____ Infant is not breathing

2. _____ Blood pressure falls profoundly

3. _____ Infant will not resume breathing on his or her own

4. _____ Heart rate falls

5. _____ Infant will resume breathing on his or her own

6. _____ Can occur in utero

A. Primary apnea

B. Secondary apnea

True/False

Use a **T** or **F** to show whether each statement is **true** or **false**.

7. _____ During secondary apnea, exposure to oxygen and stimulation usually will bring about respirations.

8. _____ An infant subjected to fetal hypoxia may go through primary apnea and into secondary apnea while in utero.

9. _____ Once an infant is in secondary apnea, even a very short delay in starting ventilation can result in a very long delay in establishing spontaneous and regular respirations.

10. _____ When an infant is apneic at birth, it usually is easy to tell whether the baby is in primary or secondary apnea.

11. _____ With progressive asphyxia, myocardial function fails and cardiac output falls.

12. _____ Delivery of an asphyxiated infant can often be anticipated on the basis of the antepartum and the intrapartum histories.

13. _____ A full set of resuscitation equipment should be present in the delivery room only when the need for resuscitation is anticipated.

14. _____ The longer an infant is allowed to go without resuscitation, the more difficult the resuscitation becomes.

15. _____ The individuals resuscitating an infant must be able to coordinate their efforts as a team.

16. _____ Personnel capable of completely and adequately resuscitating an infant should be present during every delivery.

17. _____ Neonatal resuscitation is a procedure in which the same actions are carried out regardless of the response of the infant.

18. _____ How quickly fetal lung fluid is cleared from the alveoli depends on the forcefulness of the first few breaths.

19. _____ Decisions regarding the initiation of resuscitation should be based on the 1-minute Apgar score.

20. _____ Pulmonary blood flow must increase following delivery in order for proper oxygenation to occur.

Fill In

List the ABCs of resuscitation.

21. A: _____

22. B: _____

23. C: _____

24–26. Evaluation of an infant's condition is primarily based on what three signs?

• _____

• _____

• _____

Lesson 1 Posttest: Answers

Check your answers with those given here.

Matching

1. A, B

2. B

3. B

4. A, B

5. A

6. A, B

True/False

7. **False** — This is true of *primary* apnea. An infant in *secondary* apnea is unresponsive to stimulation.

8. **True**

9. **True**

10. **False** — Primary and secondary apnea are very difficult to distinguish from one another in a clinical situation.

11. **True**

12. **True**

13. **False** — The equipment should be in the delivery room, removed from the packages and ready for use, in *every* delivery.

14. **True**

15. **True**

16. **True**

17. **False** — The flow of a resuscitation is based on the response of the infant to any particular action.

18. **True**

19. **False** — The Apgar score should not be used to determine the need to initiate resuscitation.

20. **True**

Fill In

21. A: Establish an open *airway*

22. B: Initiate *breathing*

23. C: Maintain *circulation*

24–26. • Respirations
   • Heart rate
   • Color

Decision

If . . .	Then . . .
You had at least 24 of the items correct . . .	Congratulations! You have successfully completed this posttest. Review any points that still may not be clear.
You missed 3 or more answers . . .	Review thoroughly the information regarding each item you missed. If you have any questions, see your instructor or supervisor. When you feel you have mastered all the necessary information, take the posttest again.

Appendix:
Neonatal Resuscitation Supplies and Equipment

Suction Equipment

Bulb syringe
Mechanical suction
Suction catheters 5 (or 6), 8, 10 Fr.
8 Fr. feeding tube and 20-cc syringe
Meconium aspirator

Bag-and-Mask Equipment

Infant resuscitation bag with a pressure-release valve or pressure gauge — the
    bag must be capable of delivering 90–100% oxygen
Face masks — newborn and premature sizes (cushioned rim masks preferred)
Oral airways — newborn and premature sizes
Oxygen with flowmeter and tubing

Intubation Equipment

Laryngoscope with straight blades — No. 0 (premature) and No. 1 (newborn)
Extra bulbs and batteries for laryngoscope
Endotracheal tubes — sizes 2.5, 3.0, 3.5, 4.0 mm
Stylet
Scissors
Gloves

Medications

Epinephrine 1:10,000 — 3-cc or 10-cc ampules
Naloxone hydrochloride 0.4 mg/ml — 1-ml ampules, or 1.0 mg/ml — 2-ml
    ampules
Volume expander — one or more of these:
    — Albumin 5% solution
    — Normal saline
    — Ringer's lactate
Sodium bicarbonate 4.2% (5 mEq/10 cc) — 10-cc ampules
Dextrose 10% — 250 cc
Sterile water — 30 cc
Normal saline — 30 cc

Miscellaneous

Infant resuscitation manikin
Intubation head (Lesson 5 only)
Radiant warmer
Stethoscope
Cardiotachometer with ECG oscilloscope (desirable)
Adhesive tape — 1/2- or 3/4-inch width
Syringes — 1 cc, 3 cc, 5 cc, 10 cc, 20 cc, 50 cc
Needles — 25, 21, 18
Alcohol sponges
Umbilical artery catheterization tray
Umbilical tape
Umbilical catheters 3 1/2, 5 Fr.
3-way stopcocks
5 Fr. feeding tube

Initial Steps in Resuscitation

Lesson 2

Contents

Initial Steps in Resuscitation

Lesson 2

Introduction

This lesson describes the initial steps in resuscitating a newborn infant. These steps will enable you to quickly identify infants who require resuscitation. Appropriate interventions can then be instituted without delay. The initial steps are:

- *Prevent heat loss.*
- *Clear the airway* by positioning and suctioning.
- *Initiate breathing* if necessary.
- *Evaluate the infant.*

The use of free-flow oxygen for an infant who does not need ventilation will also be discussed.

Prerequisites

The skills listed below will not be taught in this lesson but are necessary in order to perform correctly the initial steps in resuscitation. Therefore, before beginning this lesson, be sure you are able to:

- Identify neonates with central cyanosis.
- Use a bulb syringe to suction an infant's mouth and nose.
- Use a stethoscope to count a neonate's heart rate.
- Preheat the radiant warmer used by your hospital.

Objectives

When you complete this lesson, you will be able to:

Knowledge

- Recall, in correct sequence, the initial steps in resuscitation of a neonate.
- Identify illustrations that demonstrate correct positioning of the infant.
- Identify the forms of tactile stimulation that are appropriate to use for an apneic infant.
- Determine when free-flow oxygen is indicated for a newborn and list three acceptable ways to provide the oxygen.
- Describe the treatment an infant should receive if the amniotic fluid is meconium stained.
- When given a case situation, write the next immediate action to be taken or question to be answered.
- Identify statements regarding the initial steps in resuscitation as true or false.

Performance

You will also be able to:

- Successfully perform, on an infant manikin, the initial steps in resuscitation, demonstrating the ability to perform the procedures, make correct decisions, and take appropriate action based upon those decisions. The performance checklist at the end of this lesson will be used to judge your performance.

Decision Table

If ...	Then ...
You feel you can pass a test on the objectives ...	Turn to the posttest.
You wish to know more before trying the posttest ...	Go on to the next page and begin the lesson.

Glossary

The terms below are ones that you will need to know in order to understand this lesson. They are presented so that you will be familiar with them when you encounter them later.

Aspiration

The inhaling of fluid or secretions into the trachea or lungs, as shown below.

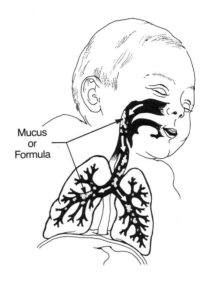

Mucus
or
Formula

Cyanosis

A bluish discoloration of the skin and mucous membranes resulting from lack of oxygen in the tissues.

Peripheral Cyanosis—Cyanosis of only the hands and feet and not the remainder of the body or mucous membranes. This results from decreased blood flow to the extremities and is normal in the initial period after birth. It is also referred to as acrocyanosis.

Central Cyanosis—Cyanosis involving the entire body, including the mucous membranes. It results from decreased oxygen in the blood.

When the term *cyanosis* is used in this lesson, it refers to *central cyanosis.*

Nares

The openings into the nose.

Nasopharynx

The part of the pharynx behind the nasal cavity and above the soft palate.

Oropharynx

The part of the pharynx between the soft palate and the upper edge of the epiglottis.

Hypopharynx

The part of the pharynx between the upper edge of the epiglottis and the openings of the larynx and esophagus.

Posterior Pharynx

Commonly referred to as the back of the throat, includes the posterior portion of the lower part of the nasopharynx and the posterior portions of the oropharynx and the hypopharynx.

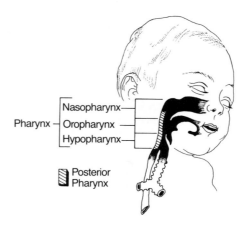

Tracheal Suctioning

Suctioning directly from the trachea, using a laryngoscope to view the trachea.

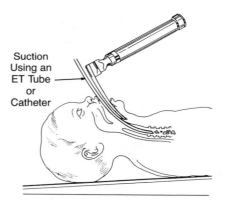

Overview of Lesson 2

Immediately after delivery, you should first place the infant under a radiant warmer and then dry him or her thoroughly to prevent heat loss. Subsequent resuscitation follows the classic *ABC* pattern:

A—Open the *airway*
B—Initiate *breathing*
C—Assure *circulation*

In this lesson, we're going to review the first steps to be taken in managing every newborn infant—even one who does not require resuscitation. We will first present the sequence for most babies, followed later in the lesson by a discussion of the additional steps necessary for a baby born with thick or particulate meconium in the amniotic fluid.

Initial Steps

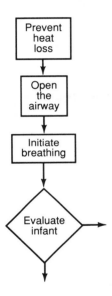

The initial steps, which can be completed within 20 seconds, are:
• Prevent heat loss

  Place the infant under a radiant heat source and dry off the amniotic fluid.
• Open the airway

  Position the infant correctly (to assure that the airway is open), and suction the infant's mouth and nose.
• Initiate breathing

  If an infant is not breathing, tactile stimulation (slapping the infant's foot or rubbing the back) is usually sufficient to stimulate respirations.

Then, we will:
• Evaluate the infant's condition

  Observe respirations, heart rate, and color to decide what further steps need to be taken.

Now let's take a look at these steps.

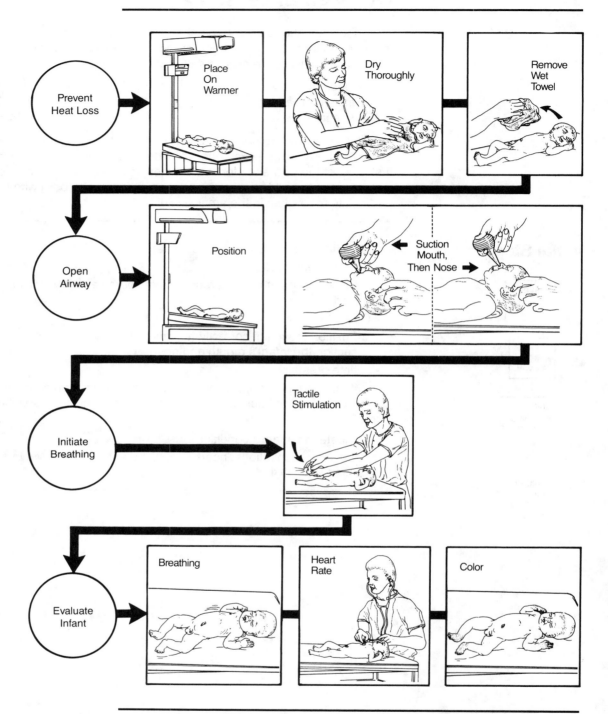

Let's begin our discussion by looking at the prevention of heat loss in a newborn infant. Then we will go into the actual resuscitation.

Preventing Heat Loss

Place Infant
on Heated
Radiant Warmer
and Dry Him
or Her

To avoid the metabolic problems brought on by cold stress, the first step in the management of the newborn infant is to prevent the loss of body heat. This can be an especially critical factor in a newborn who needs resuscitation. Heat loss is prevented by:

• Placing the infant under a radiant heat source, and
• Quickly drying him or her of amniotic fluid.

Importance

These two steps, which are appropriate for all infants following delivery, require only a few seconds to accomplish and are especially important in the case of an asphyxiated infant. Delivery rooms are usually cool to provide comfort for the mother and staff. Without proper attention to thermal management, the neonate can easily become cold stressed due to evaporative, convective, and radiant heat losses.

Even healthy, term infants are limited in their ability to produce heat when exposed to a cold environment, particularly during the first 12 hours of life. This ability is diminished even further in infants who are asphyxiated. It has been found that infants who suffer heat loss have an increased metabolic rate and require more oxygen — factors that can create serious problems for infants who already suffer asphyxia.

Using a Radiant Warmer

An overhead radiant heater provides a suitable thermal environment that minimizes radiant and convective heat loss. It is important to preheat the radiant warmer so that the infant is placed on a warm mattress.

A radiant warmer allows access to and full visualization of the infant. Blankets and clothing should not be used to cover the infant since they prevent the radiant heat waves from reaching the skin.

Drying the Infant

As soon as an infant is placed on the radiant warmer, the body and head should be quickly dried to remove amniotic fluid and to prevent evaporative heat loss. It is preferable to dry the infant with a prewarmed towel or blanket. The act of drying has a second benefit: it provides gentle stimulation, which may initiate or help maintain respirations.

Care should be taken to remove the wet towel or blanket from contact with the infant; otherwise, evaporative heat loss will continue.

Opening the Airway

Once the infant has been placed under a preheated radiant warmer and dried, the next step is to assure the "A" of our ABCs — the establishment of an open airway. This is accomplished by:

Positioning the infant correctly, and

Suctioning the infant's mouth and then nose to clear the airway.

We will examine these steps individually, beginning with positioning the infant.

Positioning

The neonate should be placed on his or her back or side with the neck slightly extended. A slight Trendelenburg position may be helpful.

CORRECT

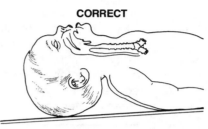

Neck Slightly Extended

Care should be taken to prevent hyperextension or underextension of the neck since either may decrease air entry.

INCORRECT

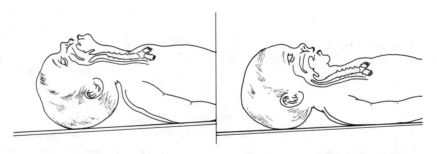

Neck Hyperextended   Neck Underextended

Shoulder Roll

To help maintain the correct position, you may place a rolled blanket or towel under the shoulders, elevating them ¾ to 1 inch off the mattress. This shoulder roll may be particularly useful if the infant has a large occiput resulting from molding, edema, or prematurity.

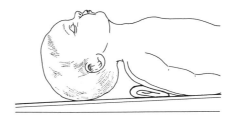

If the baby is correctly positioned, he or she is in the best position to maintain an open airway. In addition, the infant is in the optimal position for using a resuscitation bag and mask, should this become necessary.

Turning Head

If the infant has copious secretions coming from the mouth, you may want to turn the head to the side. This will allow secretions to collect in the mouth, where they can be easily removed, rather than in the posterior pharynx.

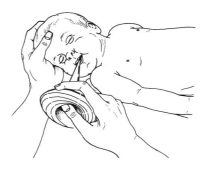

Practice

Practice positioning the manikin as described, both with and without the shoulder roll.

• Is there only a *slight* extension of the neck?

Also practice turning the head to the side.

• Can you maintain *slight* extension of the neck?

You may also find it helpful to practice in the nursery, positioning infants of various sizes.

Suctioning

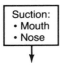

Suction:
• Mouth
• Nose

As soon as an infant has been positioned, the mouth and nose should be suctioned. The mouth is suctioned first in order to make sure that there is nothing for the infant to aspirate if he or she should gasp when the nose is suctioned.

The very act of suctioning provides a degree of *tactile stimulation.* In some cases, this is all the stimulation that is needed to initiate respirations in the infant.

If material in the mouth and nose is not removed before the infant establishes respirations, it can be aspirated into the trachea and lungs. When this occurs, the respiratory consequences can be serious.

You can use a bulb syringe or mechanical suction to remove material. Regardless of what is used, the *mouth* should be suctioned first.

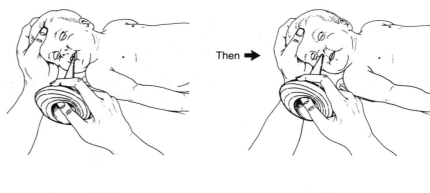

Then ➡

Mouth   Nose

Caution:

As you suction the mouth, be careful how vigorously you suction and how deep the suction catheter or bulb syringe is inserted. Stimulation of the posterior pharynx during the first few minutes after birth can produce a vagal response causing severe bradycardia and/or apnea. In healthy infants, gentle suctioning with a bulb syringe is usually adequate to remove secretions.

When using a mechanical suction apparatus, the suction pressure should be set so that when the suction tubing is occluded, the negative pressure does not exceed 100 mm Hg or 4 inches Hg.

Practice

With the manikin properly positioned, use a bulb syringe to practice suctioning the mouth and then the nose.

Summary

Let's quickly review the key steps that should be included in the process of opening the airway. Remember that this begins just as soon as the infant has been placed under a radiant warmer and dried with a towel.

1. Position the infant:
   • In a slight Trendelenburg position,
   • With the neck slightly extended.
2. Suction the mouth.
3. Suction the nose.

Practice Activity 1

The items in this practice activity are designed to help you check your understanding of the key points in the material you have read thus far. Follow the directions for each part.

Fill In

Respond to each item below by filling in the correct answer.

1. After a baby is born, he or she is placed under a radiant warmer to help protect thermal stability. What additional action would you take to assure minimal heat loss?

_____

Selection

Select the illustrations that show the infant *correctly positioned* and those that show *incorrect positioning.*

2–7. _____ Correct Positioning

_____ Incorrect Positioning

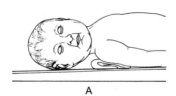

A

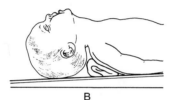

B

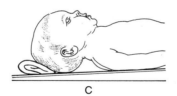

C

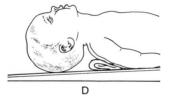

D

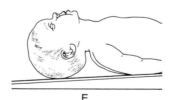

E

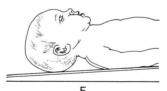

F

True/False

Use **T** or **F** to show whether a statement is **true** or **false.**

8. _____ You should not take the time to dry amniotic fluid off infants who need to be resuscitated.

9. _____ Use of a radiant warmer allows free access to the infant and at the same time provides a suitable thermal environment.

10. _____ The mattress of the radiant warmer should be preheated.

11. _____ Correct positioning of an infant is necessary for establishing an open airway.

12. _____ When infants lose heat following delivery, their metabolic rate and oxygen needs decrease.

13. _____ Stimulation of the posterior pharynx during the first few minutes after birth can produce a vagal response.

14. _____ The nose of a newborn should be suctioned first in order to facilitate breathing.

15. _____ A vagal response can lead to decreased heart rate and apnea.

16. _____ Vigorous suctioning of the posterior pharynx is recommended, as this tends to stimulate breathing.

Sequence

17. Below is a set of activities in the first part of the procedure for establishing an open airway. Number the activities according to the sequence in which they should be performed. Use 1 for the first activity, 2 for the second, etc. Assume that you have just received the infant from the delivering physician.

    _____ Position infant

    _____ Suction mouth

    _____ Dry infant

    _____ Place infant on a preheated mattress under radiant heat source

    _____ Suction nose

Practice Activity 1: Answers

Compare your responses with the ones given below. Review the material in the text that covers any items that gave you difficulty.

Fill In

1. Dry the amniotic fluid off the infant.

Selection

2–7. A, D, E — Correct Positioning

B, C, F — Incorrect Positioning

(**B** — Neck is hyperextended, shoulder roll is too high.)

(**C** — Neck is underextended, shoulder roll is improperly placed.)

(**F** — Neck is underextended.)

True/False

8. False — It is particularly important to prevent heat loss in infants who are asphyxiated.

9. True

10. True

11. True

12. False — When infants lose heat, there is an *increase* in the metabolic rate and oxygen requirement.

13. True

14. False — The mouth should be suctioned first — to make sure that there is nothing for the infant to aspirate if he or she should gasp when the nose is suctioned.

15. True

16. False — Vigorous suctioning can stimulate a vagal response, leading to severe bradycardia and/or apnea.

Sequence

17. 3 — Position infant

4 — Suction mouth

2 — Dry infant

1 — Place infant on a preheated mattress under radiant heat source

5 — Suction nose

Decision

If . . .	Then . . .
You answered at least 16 items correctly . . .	Well done! Go on to the next page and continue the good work.
You had trouble with 2 or more questions . . .	Review this section or see your instructor. Then continue with the next page.

Providing Tactile Stimulation

Provide
Tactile
Stimulation

Both drying and suctioning the infant produce stimulation, which for many infants is enough to induce respiration. If, however, an infant doesn't immediately breathe, additional tactile stimulation can be provided in an attempt to *initiate* respirations. There are two safe and appropriate methods of doing this:

- Slapping or flicking the soles of the feet, and
- Rubbing the infant's back.

Appropriate Actions

Foot Slap or Flick

Stimulating the soles of the feet, either by slapping or flicking the feet, often initiates respirations in the mildly depressed infant.

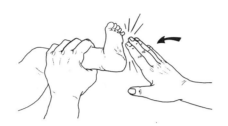
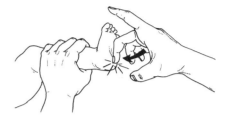

Slapping the Sole of the Foot   Flicking the Heel

Back Rub

Quickly and firmly rubbing the infant's back is another safe method of attempting to initiate respirations.

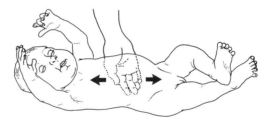

Rubbing the Infant's Back

Harmful Actions

There are certain actions, which have been used in the past to provide tactile stimulation to apneic neonates, that can harm a baby and should never be used.

Harmful Actions	Potential Consequences
• Slapping the back	Bruising
• Squeezing the rib cage	Fractures, pneumothorax, respiratory distress, death
• Forcing thighs onto abdomen	Rupture of liver or spleen, hemorrhage
• Dilating anal sphincter	Tearing of anal sphincter
• Using hot or cold compresses or baths	Hypothermia, hyperthermia, burns
• Blowing cold oxygen or air onto face or body	Hypothermia

No More
Than Twice

One or two slaps or flicks to the soles of the feet or rubbing the back once or twice will usually stimulate breathing in an infant with primary apnea. However, if the infant remains apneic, tactile stimulation should be abandoned and positive-pressure ventilation initiated immediately.

Continued use of tactile stimulation in an infant who does not respond is not warranted and may be harmful, since time is being wasted.

Gentle Rubbing

Gentle rubbing of the trunk, extremities, or head also produces tactile sensations. It is a lighter form of cutaneous stimulation than flicking or slapping the soles of the feet or firmly rubbing the back. It therefore should not be used to *initiate* respirations in an apneic infant. It can be helpful in *supporting early respiratory efforts.* Infants with respiratory effort frequently increase the rate and depth of respirations in response to gentle rubbing.

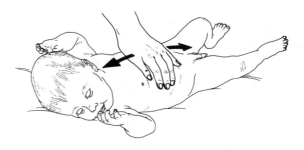

Practice

Although the steps presented so far are simple, practice performing them quickly in the correct sequence. Then you will be able to carry them out automatically at an actual delivery.

On a manikin or doll, quickly do the following:

- Place on radiant warming table (or table top for practice)
- Wipe fluid from body and head
  - Remove towel
- Quickly position
  - On back
  - Slight Trendelenburg
  - Neck slightly extended
  - Roll under shoulders (optional)
- Suction mouth, then
- Suction nose
- Provide tactile stimulation
  - Slap/flick feet, or
  - Rub back

Repeat the above steps several times until you can perform them smoothly without stopping to think, "What's next?"

Can you carry them out within 20 seconds? Time yourself.

Practice Activity 2

Now respond to these items dealing with tactile stimulation.

True/False

1. _____ Usually the stimulation of drying and suctioning an infant will start the baby breathing.

2. _____ An alternative to slapping the heel as a means of initiating respiration is to gently squeeze the rib cage.

3. _____ If there is no response to rubbing the infant's back, additional tactile stimulation should be provided by slapping or flicking the soles of the feet.

4. _____ Gentle rubbing of an infant's chest or extremities is appropriate stimulation for an apneic infant.

Selection

Which of the following actions are *harmful* and *not appropriate for tactile stimulation?*

5–9. _____

   A. Suction mouth

   B. Slap sole of foot

   C. Squeeze rib cage

   D. Apply a cold compress

   E. Force thighs onto abdomen

   F. Flick sole of foot

   G. Dilate anal sphincter

   H. Rub back

   I. Blow oxygen onto face

Case History

Read the following case history, then complete the exercise given below.

After 6 hours of labor, Mrs. Tapia gives birth to a baby boy. The baby is immediately placed under a radiant warmer, and the warmer is then turned on. Next, the infant is positioned on his back, in slight Trendelenburg with his neck hyperextended. His nose is suctioned, and then his mouth. Baby Tapia is then given tactile stimulation by slapping his foot.

10–13. List the errors ("mistakes" or "problems") in the clinical management of the infant, then state what the correct action should have been.

Error	Correct Action
_____	_____
_____	_____
_____	_____
_____	_____
_____	_____

Practice Activity 2: Answers

Here are the answers to the items on tactile stimulation.

True/False

1. True

2. False — Squeezing the rib cage can result in such complications as fracture, pneumothorax, respiratory distress, and even death.

3. False — Tactile stimulation under these circumstances would be a waste of precious time. Positive-pressure ventilation should be started immediately.

4. False — It is too gentle a form of stimulation to be used in an *apneic* baby. In a breathing infant, with respiratory effort, it can be used to increase the rate and depth of respirations.

Selection

5–9. C, D, E, G, I

Case History

10–13. Error	**Correct Action**
Radiant warmer turned on *after* baby was placed under it.	The radiant warmer should have been turned on and heated *before* the anticipated time of delivery.
Infant not dried.	The infant should be thoroughly dried of amniotic fluid as soon as possible in order to minimize heat loss by evaporation.
Neck hyperextended.	Neck should be slightly extended.
Mouth suctioned *after* the infant's nose.	The *mouth* should be suctioned *first* to prevent aspiration of any secretions when nose is suctioned.

Decision

If . . .	**Then . . .**
You had 11 items correct . . .	You're doing fine! Proceed to the next part.
You missed more than 2 . . .	Carefully review the information given for each item that gave you difficulty. When you are satisfied that you have gained the appropriate knowledge, go on to the next page.

Evaluating the Infant

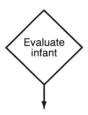

Positioning, suctioning, and stimulating are necessary in every infant at birth and are carried out to clear the airway and to initiate respirations. The next step in the resuscitation process will depend on your evaluation of the infant. You should evaluate the infant on the basis of three vital signs:

- Respiratory effort
- Heart rate
- Color

Monitoring and evaluating these signs will give you the information you need to determine what further action is appropriate.

Steps in the Evaluation

In monitoring and evaluating the infant, you generally will go through the following steps:

- Observe and evaluate the infant's respirations. If normal, go on to the next sign. If not, begin positive-pressure ventilation.
- Check the baby's heart rate. If above 100 beats/minute, go on. If not, initiate positive-pressure ventilation.
- If the infant is breathing and the heart rate is above 100, evaluate the infant's color. If central cyanosis is present, administer oxygen.

We will now briefly discuss each of these vital signs.

Respiratory Effort

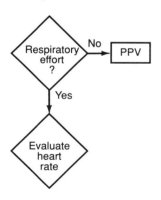

The first item to be evaluated is the infant's respiratory effort. Adequate oxygenation of the infant (resulting in sufficient oxygen for the heart and tissues and for good color) primarily depends upon adequate respirations. The rate and depth of respirations should increase in the first few seconds after the first slap or flick of the foot or rub of the back. If there is no immediate response, a second slap or flick on the sole of the foot or rub of the back may provide the necessary stimulation. Time should not be taken to stimulate the baby more than twice.

After stimulating the infant, the main question to ask is:

"Does the infant show respiratory effort?"

Breathing—If there are adequate spontaneous respirations, go on to the next step, which is to check the heart rate.

Apneic/gasping—Infants who are apneic or have gasping respirations after stimulation should be given positive-pressure ventilation (PPV). Continued tactile stimulation of an infant who is not responding only increases hypoxia and delays initiation of vitally needed ventilation. (Positive-pressure ventilation can be given with a bag and mask or with a bag and an endotracheal tube.)

Heart Rate

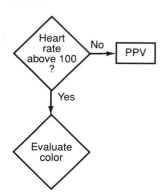

As soon as respiratory effort has been evaluated (and appropriate action taken, if needed) it is important to monitor the baby's heart rate. Don't assume that the presence of respirations will always mean that the infant has a good heart rate. Respirations may be present but may not provide adequate oxygenation to sustain a heart rate above 100 beats/minute. You will want to ask:

"Is the heart rate above or below 100?"

If the heart rate is above 100, and the infant has spontaneous respirations, you can go on to evaluate the next sign—color.

Anytime the heart rate is below 100, positive-pressure ventilation (PPV) is indicated, even though the infant may have spontaneous respirations.

Heart Rate

Below 100	Above 100
Positive-pressure ventilation	*If* spontaneous respirations, evaluate color

Note:

Monitoring the infant's heart rate is important because it often will dictate the extent of the resuscitation. From the heart rate you can determine whether positive-pressure ventilation, chest compressions, and/or the administration of medications is indicated.

If the heart rate is above 100 beats/minute and remains there, the next step is to evaluate color.

The heart rate can be checked either by using a stethoscope or by palpating the pulse in the umbilical cord or brachial artery. Palpation has the advantage of allowing continuous monitoring of the infant's heart rate.

Color

When the infant's respirations and heart rate improve significantly, the skin should also begin to turn pink. This improvement in color is due to increased oxygen entering the blood.

In some circumstances, even though the infant's respirations are adequate and the heart rate is above 100 beats/minute, the infant may still be cyanotic (central cyanosis). In this case, there is enough oxygen crossing the lungs and entering the bloodstream to sustain the heart rate, but there is not enough to fully oxygenate the infant. Under these circumstances, oxygen must be provided.

"Is cyanosis present?"

If central cyanosis is present in an infant with spontaneous respirations and an adequate heart rate, free-flow oxygen should be given.

Oxygen is not necessary for infants who have blue extremities only (peripheral cyanosis) — a condition that is present in most infants the first few minutes after birth. Peripheral cyanosis is caused by a combination of a cool delivery room and initially sluggish circulation. It is not due to a lack of oxygen.

Summary

The entire process to this point, including drying the infant, clearing the airway, and providing initial stimulation, should take no more than 20 seconds. If the infant is not breathing or the heart rate is less than 100 beats/minute, indicating inadequate respirations, it is essential to establish respirations with positive-pressure ventilation in order to assure adequate oxygenation.

Administering free-flow oxygen or continuing to provide tactile stimulation to a non-breathing infant or to one whose heart rate is below 100 beats/minute is of little or no value and only delays appropriate management.

Practice Activity 3

Here are some questions about evaluating a newborn infant. Give each item your careful consideration, then write your response.

Fill In

List, in the sequence in which they should be obtained, the three signs used to evaluate each newborn.

1. _____

2. _____

3. _____

4. While you are suctioning and stimulating an infant, you observe no respiratory movement. Why should you immediately initiate positive-pressure ventilation rather than continue tactile stimulation?

_____

_____

_____

5. A new infant has a respiratory response to tactile stimulation. You should expect that within 15–30 seconds, the heart rate should be above

_____.

True/False

6. _____ If an infant is breathing, you can be sure that the heart rate is above 100.

7. _____ An infant's heart rate often serves as an indicator of the extent of the needed resuscitation.

8. _____ The Apgar score should be used as the indicator of a neonate's need for resuscitation.

Case Situation

9. You find that an infant makes no respiratory movement after suctioning and tactile stimulation. What action should be taken?

_____

10. Baby Lewis is apneic at birth, but after suctioning, some respiratory movement is noted. You slap the infant's foot twice but the infant does not establish adequate respirations. What is your next appropriate action?

_____

_____

_____

11. A newborn infant has been positioned, suctioned, provided with tactile stimulation, and you have evaluated his or her respirations as normal. What is the next step in your evaluation?

   _____

12. Your evaluation of an infant shows that both respirations and heart rate are satisfactory, but the baby has central cyanosis. What action should you take?

   _____

13. After providing tactile stimulation, you find that an infant is breathing but the heart rate is 90 beats/minute. What action should be taken?

   _____

Practice Activity 3: Answers

Check your answers carefully against the ones given here. Review the text content for any items that may have given you difficulty.

Fill In

1. Respiratory effort

2. Heart rate

3. Color

4. The infant may be too depressed (as in secondary apnea) to respond to tactile stimulation. Positive-pressure ventilation is probably required to initiate respirations.

5. 100

True/False

6. **False** — Even though respirations are present, they may not be strong enough to sustain a heart rate above 100.

7. **True**

8. **False** — The first Apgar score is generally not determined until 1 minute after birth. In many cases resuscitation should be started *before* this time.

Case Situation

9. Initiate positive-pressure ventilation

10. Begin positive-pressure ventilation

11. Evaluate the baby's heart rate

12. Administer free-flow oxygen

13. Begin positive-pressure ventilation

Decision

If . . .	Then . . .
You had the correct answers to at least 12 of the 13 items . . .	Good work! Go right on to the next page.
You missed 2 or more . . .	Review the text material related to each item you missed. If you have questions, see your instructor before going on.

Use of Free-Flow Oxygen

At birth, most infants have some degree of cyanosis. As respirations are established, oxygenation improves so that by 60–90 seconds, most infants are beginning to become pink, although peripheral cyanosis may still be present.

There are times, however, when an infant has established regular respirations and the heart rate is above 100 beats/minute, but central cyanosis persists. In such cases, the respirations may be adequate to provide enough oxygen to keep the heart rate above 100, but not adequate to fully oxygenate the infant. Persistent cyanosis can also be due to a congenital defect that interferes with pulmonary function (e.g., diaphragmatic hernia) or congenital heart disease.

To relieve cyanosis in **infants with adequate respirations and a heart rate above 100 beats/minute, free-flow oxygen should be given to improve the color. Positive-pressure ventilation is not indicated.**

Principles

Here you will learn how to manage free-flow oxygen:
• Initially,
• Once the infant becomes pink, and
• If cyanosis persists.

Initially

A newborn infant who has central cyanosis *after* respirations are established and a heart rate above 100, should initially receive a high concentration of oxygen—at least 80%.

When Pink

Once the infant becomes pink, the oxygen should be *gradually* withdrawn, until the infant can remain pink while breathing room air, as clinically appropriate.

When Cyanosis Persists

Infants who become cyanotic as the oxygen is withdrawn should continue to receive just enough oxygen to remain pink—and no more.

Free-Flow Oxygen

Free-flow oxygen refers to blowing oxygen over the infant's nose so that the infant breathes oxygen-enriched air.

For a brief time, this can be accomplished by using
• Oxygen tubing
• Oxygen mask
• Anesthesia bag and mask

Actual Concentration of Oxygen

Your wall or portable oxygen source sends 100% oxygen through the tubing. As oxygen flows from the tubing, it mixes with room air. The concentration of oxygen that reaches the infant's nose is determined by the amount of 100% oxygen coming from the tube (stated in liter flow per minute) and the amount of room air it must pass through to reach the infant. Room air contains 21% oxygen. Thus, when 100% oxygen is mixed with room air, the concentration of oxygen reaching the infant is less than 100%.

Oxygen Tubing

In those circumstances where a specific concentration of oxygen is necessary you must set the correct combination of:

- Liter flow, and
- Distance from the end of the tube to the infant's nose.

The concentration can be controlled with a flow of 5 liters/minute. The closer the tubing is to the nose, the higher the concentration delivered. The infant receives the maximum amount of oxygen (approximately 80%) when the tube is one-half inch from the nose. Withdrawing the tube 1 or 2 inches causes a rapid fall in oxygen concentration.

The tubing should be held *steady* and aimed at the nares. Waving the end of the tubing back and forth in front of the nose decreases the oxygen concentration considerably.

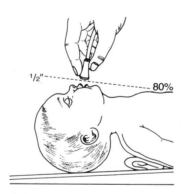

Oxygen Mask

If you are using tubing with an oxygen mask attached and the oxygen flow is 5 liters per minute, you can deliver a high concentration of oxygen by holding the mask *firmly* on the baby's face.

Mask Held Firmly

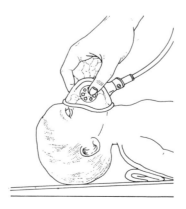

Anesthesia Bag and Mask

As you will learn in the next lesson, an anesthesia bag and mask, when attached to an oxygen source, can also be used to deliver high concentrations of free-flow oxygen.

Caution in the Use of Oxygen

Remember that you must provide enough oxygen for the infant to become pink. After the resuscitation, once you have established the infant on oxygen, immediately move him or her into an area where choice of O_2 concentration (FiO_2) can be based on blood gas (PaO_2) values.

To prevent heat loss and drying of the respiratory mucosa, oxygen given neonates should be heated and humidified. However, during an emergency, dry oxygen may be given *briefly* to stabilize the infant's condition. If oxygen is to be continued for more than a few minutes, it should be heated and humidified. When oxygen is heated and humidified, it must be provided via wide-bore tubing.

Practice Activity 4

The items in this practice activity will allow you to test your knowledge of the key concepts in administering free-flow oxygen to neonates.

Fill In

1. What concentration of oxygen should you initially provide an infant who is breathing without assistance, whose heart rate is above 100, and who is cyanotic?

   _____

2. When providing oxygen to a neonate using an oxygen tube or oxygen mask, what setting should you use for the flowmeter?

   _____ liters/minute

True/False

3. _____ When oxygen is used with infants for more than a few minutes, it should be heated and humidified.

4. _____ If an infant who is receiving free-flow oxygen at 80% becomes pink, you should immediately turn off the flowmeter, discontinuing the oxygen.

5. _____ Waving the oxygen tubing back and forth in front of the nose provides a lower concentration of oxygen than holding the tube steady.

Selecting

Which of these illustrations shows a correct way to initially provide free-flow oxygen to an infant?

6. _____

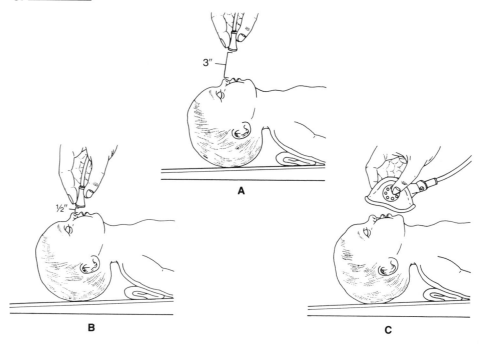

Fill In

7. What is incorrect about the techniques shown in the other illustrations above? Note the letter of the illustration and the mistakes.

Illustration _____ shows:

_____

Illustration _____ shows:

_____

Practice Activity 4: Answers

Some of the items in this practice activity required you to give specific numbers. As you check your answers, be certain that you do so carefully.

Fill In

1. At least 80%

2. 5 liters/minute

True/False

3. **True**

4. **False** — Once the infant becomes pink, the oxygen should be *gradually* withdrawn, to see if the infant can remain pink in room air, as clinically appropriate.

5. **True**

Selecting

6. Illustration **B** is correct

Fill In

7. Illustration A shows:
   - Tubing too far from nose

   Illustration C shows:
   - Mask held too far from face

Decision

If . . .	Then . . .
You were correct on at least 6 of the 7 answers . . .	You're doing well! Please go on to the next page.
You missed 2 or more items . . .	Review the text material for those items. See your instructor if you have any questions.

Meconium in Amniotic Fluid

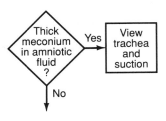

It is extremely important to observe whether meconium is present in the amniotic fluid. When meconium has been expelled into the amniotic fluid, there is a chance the meconium will be aspirated into the infant's mouth and potentially into the trachea and lungs. Appropriate steps must be taken during and immediately following the delivery in an attempt to prevent serious consequences resulting from aspiration of the meconium.

Thin, Watery

Small amounts of meconium passed by the fetus well before delivery may merely discolor the amniotic fluid, with *no particles* of meconium visible. Such fluid is often described as thin or watery meconium-stained fluid. Special management of these infants is probably not necessary.

Thick, Particulate

The following steps refer to those infants in whom the amniotic fluid contains thick meconium — amniotic fluid that is "pea soup" in appearance or contains particles of meconium.

Clearing the Airway of Meconium

To make certain that all thick or particulate meconium-stained fluid is cleared from the airway, suctioning should take place:
- When the head is delivered, and
- When the infant has been placed on a warmer.

When Head Is Delivered

As soon as the baby's head is delivered (before delivery of the shoulders), using a 10 Fr. or larger suction catheter:
- The mouth, pharynx, and nose should be thoroughly suctioned.

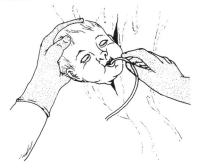

After Delivery

As soon as the infant has been placed on the radiant warmer and before drying, two steps should be taken:
- Residual meconium in the hypopharynx should be removed by suctioning under direct vision
- The trachea should then be intubated and meconium suctioned from the lower airway

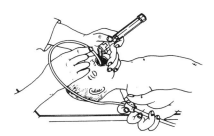

In the presence of thick meconium, this is best done by applying suction to an endotracheal tube. Once the endotracheal tube has been inserted, *continuous* suction is applied to the tube as it is withdrawn. Suction can be applied to the endotracheal tube by use of an adaptor and a regulated wall suction device.

Reintubation followed by suctioning should be repeated until returns are nearly free of meconium.

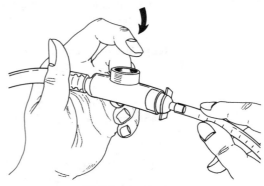

Wall Suction Device

Note:

To minimize hypoxia when suctioning under direct vision, free-flow oxygen should be provided via oxygen tubing.

After tracheal suctioning, the stomach should be suctioned to prevent aspiration of meconium-containing gastric contents. If positive-pressure ventilation is not required, wait until the infant is at least 5 minutes of age before suctioning the stomach. This will minimize the chance of producing a vagal response with apnea and bradycardia.

Caution:

Attempts should not be made to suction meconium from the trachea by passing a suction catheter *through* an endotracheal tube. The catheter size required to fit through an endotracheal tube in a newborn is too small to adequately remove meconium.

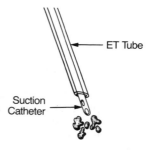

ET Tube

Suction
Catheter

When thick or particulate meconium-stained fluid is present, tracheal suctioning should be completed as soon after delivery as possible. This requires the presence of someone in the delivery room who has the capability to visualize the glottis with a laryngoscope and to suction the trachea under direct vision. Under these conditions, this task must take priority over any other assigned to this person.

Using the laryngoscope to visualize the glottis and inserting an endotracheal tube is taught in a later lesson entitled "Endotracheal Intubation."

Clinical Judgment

When managing an infant who has passed meconium in utero, clinical judgment may alter the protocol at two points.

If an infant has passed thick meconium, yet is very active and crying vigorously, a judgment must be made whether the difficulty of intubating a vigorous infant outweighs the advantages of full meconium removal. However, many experienced individuals believe that meconium removal may be of primary importance to prevent the sequelae of meconium aspiration.

In an infant with severe asphyxia, clinical judgment should be used to determine the number of reintubations. It may not be possible to clear the trachea of all meconium before initiating positive-pressure ventilations.

Responsibility

Prior to the delivery of any infant with meconium-stained fluid, it is essential to determine who will have the responsibility for laryngoscoping and suctioning the infant. You will only know whether or not meconium exists after the membranes have ruptured. Consequently, at any delivery, it is important that the proper equipment and the personnel skilled in using that equipment be on hand and ready to act instantly.

Practice Activity 5

Before completing the following items, you may want to review the text material dealing with suctioning and meconium aspiration.

True/False

Indicate whether the following statements are **true** or **false.**

1. _____ Infants with thin, watery meconium-stained amniotic fluid do not need tracheal suctioning at birth.

2. _____ If there is meconium in the amniotic fluid, it is possible for this meconium to be aspirated into the infant's lungs upon and after delivery.

3. _____ Because a laryngoscope is seldom used on a neonate, it is usually satisfactory to send for one when the need arises.

4. _____ You will always know prior to the delivery whether the amniotic fluid is meconium stained.

5. _____ The stomach should be suctioned to prevent aspiration of gastric contents containing meconium at some time after tracheal suctioning.

Case Situation

Before Baby Nelson is born, particulate meconium is observed in the amniotic fluid. Describe the special steps that should be taken in the delivery room to prevent aspiration of meconium.

6. When head is delivered:

_____

_____

7. After baby is delivered and placed under a radiant heater (two steps):

• _____

• _____

8. What might happen if meconium remained in the infant's trachea?

_____

_____

Multiple Choice

Which of the following is recommended for suctioning meconium from the *trachea?*

9. _____

A. 6 or 8 Fr. suction catheter

B. Endotracheal tube

C. Suction catheter passed through an endotracheal tube

Practice Activity 5: Answers

Use the following responses to check your answers to this practice activity. For any items missed, review the appropriate information in the lesson.

True/False

1. **True**

2. **True**

3. **False** — Any time the need for resuscitation is anticipated, both the proper equipment and the skilled personnel should be on hand during the delivery.

4. **False** — You will know only if the membranes have ruptured.

5. **True**

Case Situation

6. When the head is delivered — thoroughly suction *the mouth, pharynx, and nose.*

7. After the baby is delivered and placed under a radiant heater:
   • Suction residual meconium from hypopharynx
   • Intubate and suction trachea

8. The infant may aspirate some of the meconium into his or her lungs.

Multiple Choice

9. **B**

Decision

If . . .	Then . . .
You had *all* the items correct . . .	You evidently have a good knowledge of the key ideas associated with suctioning and meconium aspiration. Go right on to the part on tactile stimulation.
You missed 1 or more . . .	Before you go on, study again the pages containing information on the items that gave you trouble. Check with your instructor if you need help.

Summary

This summary of the initial steps in resuscitation and some guidelines for practice are presented for your review and reference.

Preventing Heat Loss

The first step in caring for a newborn is to prevent heat loss. Heat loss is prevented by:
- Placing the infant under a heated radiant warmer, and
- Quickly drying the infant of amniotic fluid.

Positioning

Next, the infant should be positioned properly to assure an open airway. For correct positioning:
- Neonate is placed on his or her back or side, in slight Trendelenburg with the neck slightly extended.

Suctioning

As soon as the infant is properly positioned, he or she should be suctioned:
- Suction the *mouth first,*
- Then suction the nose.

Tactile Stimulation

If an infant doesn't breathe immediately, tactile stimulation should be started in an attempt to initiate respirations. There are two correct methods of tactile stimulation:
- Slapping or flicking the soles of the feet, and
- Rubbing the back.

Harmful actions such as the following should be avoided:
- Slapping the back,
- Squeezing the rib cage,
- Forcing thighs onto abdomen,
- Dilating anal sphincter,
- Using hot or cold compresses or baths, and
- Blowing cold oxygen or air onto face or body.

Gentle rubbing of trunk, extremities, or head can be used to increase respiratory effort in a baby who is breathing.

Evaluation

After you have provided tactile stimulation, you should monitor and evaluate the infant on the basis of three vital signs:
- Respiratory effort,
- Heart rate, and
- Color.

You should follow these steps:

Respirations

Observe and evaluate the infant's respirations. If normal, go on to the next sign. If not, begin positive-pressure ventilation.

Heart Rate

Check the baby's heart rate. If above 100 beats/minute, go on. If not, initiate positive-pressure ventilation.

Color

Observe and evaluate infant's color. If central cyanosis is present, administer free-flow oxygen.

Meconium

If thick or particulate meconium is present in the amniotic fluid, *the obstetrician should suction the mouth, pharynx, and nose as soon as the baby's head is delivered,* prior to delivery of the shoulders.

After delivery, the hypopharynx should be suctioned to remove residual meconium, and then the trachea should be intubated and any residual meconium removed by applying continuous suction to the endotracheal tube as it is being withdrawn.

Practice

Practice sequencing all steps so they become automatic. Take the manikin and place it on the table and quickly do the following:

1. Dry thoroughly, then remove the wet towel
2. Position correctly
3. Suction mouth
4. Suction nose
5. Slap or flick feet, or rub back
6. Pretend evaluating
   - Respirations
   - Heart rate
   - Color

You should be able to complete these steps within 20 seconds. If you cannot, practice until you can do so.

How would you handle each of the following situations? The *correct* management is given on the preceding page.

Respirations

- Apneic — no respirations
- Normal respirations

Heart Rate

- Above 100
- Below 100

Color

- Infant pink
- Peripheral cyanosis — hands and feet remain blue while rest of baby is pink
- Central cyanosis — entire baby is cyanotic

Posttest
Lesson 2—Initial Steps in Resuscitation

Name _____ Date _____

This posttest is designed to test your knowledge of the key points in Lesson 2. Follow the directions for each part and give careful consideration to each question.

Selection

Select the illustrations that show the infant *correctly positioned.*

1–3. _____ Correct Positioning

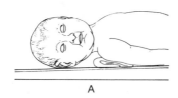

A

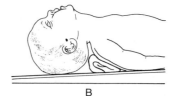

B

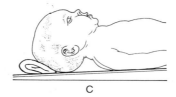

C

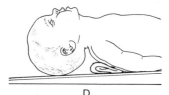

D

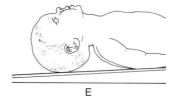

E

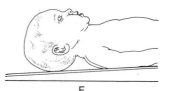

F

True/False

Use **T** or **F** to show whether a statement is **true** or **false.**

4. _____ You should not take the time to dry amniotic fluid off infants who need to be resuscitated.

5. _____ Correct positioning of an infant is necessary for establishing an open airway.

6. _____ The nose of a newborn should be suctioned first in order to facilitate breathing.

7. _____ A vagal response can lead to decreased heart rate and apnea.

Sequence

8. Below is a set of activities in the initial steps of resuscitating an infant. Indicate the correct order by numbering the activities according to the sequence in which they should be performed. Use 1 for the first activity, 2 for the second, etc. Assume that you have just been handed the infant by the delivering physician.

_____ Position infant

_____ Suction mouth

_____ Dry infant

_____ Place infant on a preheated mattress under radiant heat source

_____ Suction nose

True/False

Indicate whether the following statements are **true** or **false**.

9. _____ If there is meconium in the amniotic fluid, it is possible for this meconium to be aspirated into the infant's lungs upon and after delivery.

10. _____ You will always know prior to the delivery whether the amniotic fluid is meconium stained.

11. _____ If an infant who is receiving free-flow oxygen at 80% becomes pink, you should immediately turn off the flowmeter, discontinuing the oxygen.

Case Situation

Before Baby Nelson is born, particulate meconium is observed in the amniotic fluid. Describe the special steps that should be taken in the delivery room to prevent aspiration of meconium.

12. When the head is delivered:

• _____

13. Once the baby is delivered and placed under a radiant heater (two steps):

• _____

• _____

Multiple Choice

14. Which of the following is recommended for suctioning meconium from the _trachea?_ _____

A. Endotracheal tube

B. 6 or 8 Fr. suction catheter

C. Suction catheter passed through an endotracheal tube

True/False

15. _____ If an infant is not responding to rubbing of the back, you should continue to provide tactile stimulation by slapping or flicking the soles of the feet.

16. _____ Gentle rubbing of an infant's chest or extremities is appropriate stimulation for an apneic infant.

Selecting

Which of the following actions are *harmful* and *not appropriate* for *tactile stimulation?*

17–21. _____

A. Suction mouth

B. Slap sole of foot

C. Squeeze rib cage

D. Apply a cold compress

E. Force thighs onto abdomen

F. Flick sole of foot

G. Dilate anal sphincter

H. Rub back

I. Blow oxygen onto face

Fill In

List, in the sequence in which they should be obtained, the three signs used to evaluate each newborn.

22. _____

23. _____

24. _____

True/False

25. _____ If an infant is exhibiting any respiratory effort, you can be sure that the heart rate is above 100.

26. _____ An infant's heart rate often serves as an indicator of the extent of the needed resuscitation.

27. _____ The Apgar score should be used as the indicator of a neonate's need for resuscitation.

Case Situation

28. You find that an infant makes no respiratory movement after suctioning and tactile stimulation. What action should be taken?

_____

29. A newborn infant has been positioned, suctioned, provided with tactile stimulation, and you have evaluated his or her respirations as normal. What is the next step in your evaluation?

_____

30. Your evaluation of an infant shows that both respirations and heart rate are satisfactory, but the baby has central cyanosis. What action should you take?

_____

31. After providing tactile stimulation, you find that an infant is breathing but the heart rate is 90 beats/minute. What action should be taken?

_____

Fill In

32. What concentration of oxygen should you initially provide an infant who is breathing without assistance, whose heart rate is above 100, and who has central cyanosis?

_____

33. When providing oxygen to a neonate with an oxygen tube or oxygen mask, what setting should you use for the flowmeter?

_____ liters/minute

Selecting

34-35. Which of these illustrations show acceptable ways to provide free-flow oxygen to an infant who is breathing spontaneously?

_____

A	B	C

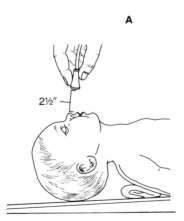 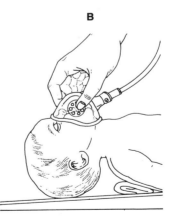 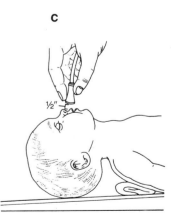

Lesson 2 Posttest: Answers

Check your answers carefully against the ones given here. Review the text material for any items that gave you difficulty.

Selection

1–3. A, D, E — Correct positioning

(Incorrect positioning:

B — Neck is hyperextended, shoulder roll is too high.

C — Neck is underextended, shoulder roll is improperly placed.

F — Neck is underextended.)

True/False

4. False — It is particularly important to prevent heat loss in infants who are asphyxiated.

5. True

6. False — The mouth should be suctioned first — to make sure that there is nothing for the infant to aspirate if he or she should gasp when the nose is suctioned.

7. True

Sequence

8. 3 — Position infant

4 — Suction mouth

2 — Dry infant

1 — Place infant on a preheated mattress under radiant heat source

5 — Suction nose

True/False

9. True

10. False — You will know only if the membranes have ruptured.

11. False — Once the infant becomes pink, the oxygen should be *gradually* withdrawn, to see if the infant can remain pink in room air, as clinically appropriate.

Case Situation

12. When the head is delivered — *thoroughly suction the mouth, pharynx, and nose.*

13. Once the baby is delivered and placed under a radiant heater:
• Suction residual meconium from hypopharynx
• Intubate and suction trachea

Multiple Choice

14. A

True/False

15. False—Tactile stimulation under these circumstances would be a waste of precious time. Positive-pressure ventilation should be started immediately.

16. False—It is too gentle a form of stimulation to be used in an *apneic* baby. In an infant with some respiratory effort, it can be used to increase the rate and depth of respirations.

Selecting

17–21. C, D, E, G, I

Fill In

22. Respiratory effort

23. Heart rate

24. Color

True/False

25. False—Even though respirations are present, they may not be adequate to sustain a heart rate above 100.

26. True

27. False—The first Apgar score is not determined until 1 minute after birth. In many cases, resuscitation should be started *before* this time.

Case Situation

28. Initiate positive-pressure ventilation — bag and mask or bag and endotracheal tube

29. Evaluate the baby's heart rate

30. Administer free-flow oxygen

31. Begin positive-pressure ventilation — bag and mask or bag and endotracheal tube

Fill In

32. At least 80%

33. 5 liters/minute

Selecting

34-35. B and **C** are correct

Decision

If . . .	Then . . .
You were correct on at least 33 of the 35 answers . . .	You've done well! Please go on and practice the initial steps using the performance checklist on the following pages.
You missed 3 or more items . . .	Review the text material that relates to those items. See your instructor if you have any questions.

Performance Checklist
Lesson 2—Initial Steps in Resuscitation

Instructions

Instructor: The participant should be instructed to talk through the procedure as it is demonstrated. Judge the performance of each step carried out, and check (✔) the box when the action is completed correctly. If done incorrectly, circle the box so that you can discuss that step later.

Present each of the situations given. This allows the participant to demonstrate the initial steps for an infant without meconium-stained amniotic fluid and for an infant with thick meconium in the amniotic fluid.

After the participant has been through the procedure twice, provide additional clinical situations if desired to ensure that the participant fully understands the procedure.

It is recommended that an infant resuscitation manikin be used for the demonstration. When a manikin is used, you must provide, at several points, information concerning the condition of the "infant." This allows you to check the participant's ability to make correct decisions and take the appropriate action based on those decisions.

To successfully complete this checklist, the participant should be able to perform *all* the steps and make correct decisions in the procedure.

Equipment and Supplies

Infant resuscitation manikin
Bulb syringe
Stethoscope
Oxygen source with flowmeter
Oxygen tubing
Shoulder roll
Blanket/towel to dry infant
Bag and mask
Laryngoscope and blade
ET tube

Performance Checklist
Lesson 2—Initial Steps in Resuscitation

Name _____ Instructor _____ Date _____

Situation One

"An infant has just been delivered. The amniotic fluid is clear. Demonstrate how you would manage the infant."

Situation Two

"An infant has just been delivered. There is thick meconium in the amniotic fluid. Demonstrate how you would proceed with the infant."

☐ **1. If there is evidence of thick or particulate, meconium-stained amniotic fluid, participant indicates he or she would request presence of someone in delivery room capable of tracheal suctioning**

Instructor: Hands newly delivered infant to participant

☐ **2. Places infant on preheated radiant warmer**

☐ **3. If thick or particulate meconium in amniotic fluid, indicates he or she would perform or request tracheal suctioning**

☐ **4. Dries amniotic fluid from body and head**

☐ **5. Removes wet linen from contact with infant**

☐ **6. Positions infant with neck slightly extended**

☐ **7. Suctions mouth, then nose**

☐ **8. Evaluates respirations**

Breathing   Apneic/gasping

☐ Slaps foot, flicks heel, or rubs back 1–2 times only

☐ Evaluates respirations

Breathing   Apneic/gasping

☐ Indicates positive-pressure ventilation needed

☐ **9. Evaluates heart rate**

Above 100   Below 100

☐ Indicates positive-pressure ventilation needed

☐ **10. Evaluates color**

Pink or peripheral cyanosis   Central cyanosis

Continues to observe infant

☐ Provides free-flow oxygen 80 -100% O_2

☐ Evaluates color

Pink   Cyanotic

☐ Slowly withdraws O_2, keeping baby barely pink

☐ Continues free-flow oxygen 80 -100% O_2

Use of a Resuscitation Bag and Mask: Equipment

Lesson 3A

Contents

Use of a Resuscitation Bag and Mask: Equipment

Overview of Lesson 3

In the previous lesson, you learned the first steps in resuscitating a neonate. If an infant does not respond immediately to clearing the airway and tactile stimulation, positive-pressure ventilation must be started promptly and performed correctly. If you intervene quickly and effectively, infants usually will respond, and you will not need to go further with the resuscitation.

Positive-pressure ventilation can be given either with a resuscitation bag and mask or a bag and endotracheal tube. We will deal with the use of the bag and mask in this lesson and the insertion of an endotracheal tube in a later lesson. The principles of ventilation, however, are the same for both.

The ability to perform safe and effective ventilation requires skill and practice. Before you can develop this skill and put it to work, there are three important things you must do:

- Get acquainted with the equipment and how it works.
- Learn how to safely ventilate an infant using a bag and mask.
- Learn where ventilation fits as part of the total resuscitation procedure.

This lesson contains the information you will need to develop the appropriate knowledge and skills for using a bag and mask to ventilate a newborn infant. This information will be divided into three parts.

Part A — Equipment

You will learn about selecting the appropriate equipment and how it works.

In Part A you will learn about the types of bags and masks generally available. You will be given information on their preferred features — ones that make them safer and easier to use. You will also learn how to assemble the equipment, and you will understand how a resuscitation bag actually works.

You must become thoroughly familiar with the equipment used where *you* work. Only then can you implement the resuscitation procedure effectively.

Part B — Ventilating the Infant

An introduction to the ventilation procedure is presented in Part B. Here you will learn how to actually use the equipment available in your hospital so you can practice bag-and-mask ventilation. You will learn how to obtain a seal with the mask and how to use the recommended rate and pressure for ventilating a newborn infant. It is important that you are able to obtain a seal with the mask quickly and ventilate at the correct rate and pressure before proceeding to the final part of the lesson.

Part C — Ventilation as Part of the Resuscitation Procedure

Here you will learn when to use bag-and-mask ventilation in resuscitating a newborn infant and the proper sequence in providing positive-pressure ventilation. Cases will be presented for testing your understanding of the procedure and of the concepts and principles involved.

Clinical Performance Checklists

A clinical performance checklist is included in both Part B and Part C. They have been provided for your use in practicing ventilation. Your instructor will use the checklists to make sure that you are able to use the equipment correctly and to perform all the steps properly and in the correct sequence. You will find that the use of an infant resuscitation manikin will be very helpful as you practice following the steps in each of the checklists.

Prerequisite

Inserting an orogastric catheter and suctioning the stomach of a newborn infant is essential to providing effective ventilation with a bag and mask. To successfully complete Lessons 3B and 3C you must be able to do this. If you cannot, discuss it with your instructor or supervisor so that arrangements can be made for you to attain this skill.

Part A Objectives

When you have completed this lesson, you will be able to:

- Correctly identify the parts of an anesthesia and/or self-inflating bag and be able to state their functions.
- State the two safety features that help control the pressure provided by resuscitation bags.
- State the concentration of oxygen delivered by resuscitation bags when assembled in various ways.
- State the criteria for proper fit of a resuscitation mask.
- Select from a group of illustrations the ones in which resuscitation masks fit and are positioned correctly.
- Identify true statements about resuscitation bags and masks.

Decision Table

If . . .	Then . . .
You feel you can pass a test on these objectives . . .	Turn to the posttest on page 3A-37.
You wish to know more before attempting the test . . .	Continue on the next page.

Equipment

This lesson will help you become familiar with the equipment you will use when ventilating an infant with a resuscitation bag and mask. Although there is a variety of equipment that can be used, in this lesson we will attempt to give you an orientation to the equipment used in *your* hospital.

Equipment Used in Your Work Area

It is important that you become completely familiar with the specific equipment used where *you* work.

In order to go through Part A of this lesson, you will need to gather specific equipment. This should include a resuscitation bag, resuscitation masks, and appropriate equipment for using oxygen with the bag.

In some hospitals, the resuscitation equipment used for neonates varies from one department or unit to another. For example, resuscitation bags used in the delivery room may be a different brand than those used in the nursery or the emergency room. The same may be true for masks or oxygen equipment. If that is true in your hospital, be certain that you select the equipment that is used in the area or areas in which you will be working. If you have any questions as to what is used or where to find it, be sure to ask your instructor or supervisor for assistance.

A summary list of the equipment you will need is given here.

Bags

Resuscitation bag or bags (if more than one type or brand is used, obtain one of each)

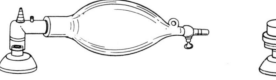
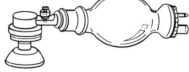

Anesthesia Bag   Self-Inflating Bag

Pressure gauge, if one is used

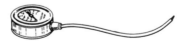

Oxygen reservoir

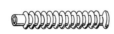
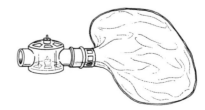

Masks

Face masks (one of each type and size used)

Oxygen Equipment

Oxygen source (oxygen tank or a wall oxygen outlet)

Flowmeter

Oxygen tubing

Air/oxygen blender, if used in your area

Manikin (optional)

For this part of the lesson, an infant resuscitation manikin is optional. It will be required for Parts B and C. If it is readily available, it would be useful with Part A.

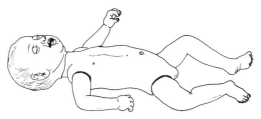

Equipment Manual

It may prove helpful to have at hand a copy of the operating manual for the resuscitation bag(s) you have.

Gather Equipment

Now, before you go any further in this lesson, stop and obtain the equipment you will need. Once you have the equipment, keep it in front of you as you work through this lesson.

Types of Bags

Before we begin to look specifically at the equipment used in your hospital, there is some information you should have about the various types of resuscitation bags available. There are two types of resuscitation bags:
- The anesthesia bag (flow-inflating bag), and
- The self-inflating bag.

Anesthesia Bag (Flow-Inflating)

The anesthesia bag is collapsed when not in use, and it looks like a deflated balloon. It inflates only when air or oxygen is forced into the bag. It therefore is dependent on a compressed gas source.

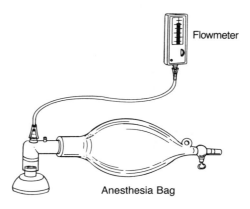

Flowmeter

Anesthesia Bag

Self-Inflating Bag

The self-inflating bag, as its name implies, inflates automatically without a compressed gas source. It remains inflated at all times, ready for use. Since it is not dependent on a compressed gas source for inflation, it is portable.

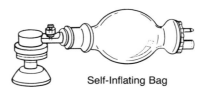

Self-Inflating Bag

Although different *brands* of each type may appear quite different from one another, each bag can be classified as either an anesthesia or a self-inflating bag. *Which* classification a bag is given depends upon its mechanism of inflation.

The anesthesia bag and the self-inflating bag will be discussed separately. You will learn more about how the bags inflate, what their basic differences are, what the safety features are, and how oxygen can be used with each.

Practice activities and exercises will provide guidelines for practice. They also will enable you to test your understanding of resuscitation bags and how they operate.

Note:

If you have an *anesthesia bag,* go right to the next page and study the material having to do with that type of bag. If you are using only a *self-inflating* bag, you do not need to read about the anesthesia bag, but can turn to page 3A-19, where the self-inflating bag is discussed. If you have *both* types of bags, it is important for you to learn how to use both. In other words, as you continue in this lesson, you should concentrate on those portions that are appropriate to the type of equipment you will be using.

Anesthesia Bag

If you will be using an anesthesia bag, this is the section you should study next.

Parts

There are two parts of an anesthesia bag that you should be able to identify:
• Gas inlet and
• Patient outlet.

Gas Inlet

The *gas inlet* is where the compressed gas enters the bag. The inlet is a small projection that is designed to fit oxygen tubing. The inlet may be at either end of the bag, depending on the brand and model you have.

Gas Inlet

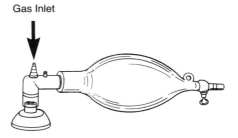

Practice

Before you go on, locate the *gas inlet* on your anesthesia bag and practice attaching the oxygen tube. (If you need any assistance or have any questions, see your instructor or supervisor.)

Patient Outlet

The *patient outlet* is where air exits from the bag to the patient. It is where the mask or endotracheal (ET) tube attaches to the bag.

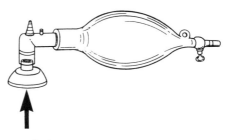

Patient Outlet

Practice

Now locate the *patient outlet* on your anesthesia bag.

Optional Parts

There are two additional parts that appear on many anesthesia bags. These are the:

- Flow-control valve and
- Pressure-gauge attachment site.

Both can create problems with inflation of the bag if you do not understand them.

**Flow-Control
Valve**

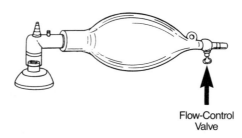

Flow-Control
Valve

The flow-control valve governs an opening that some anesthesia bags have. The opening provides an additional outlet for the compressed gas. It allows excess gas to escape rather than overinflate the bag or be forced into the patient. The size of the opening can be controlled by adjusting the flow-control valve, thereby regulating the flow of gas escaping from the bag.

Practice

Check to see whether your anesthesia bag has a *flow-control valve.* If so, how do you control flow through the valve?

**Pressure-Gauge
Attachment Site**

Anesthesia bags often have a site for attaching a pressure gauge. The attachment site is usually close to the patient outlet. The pressure gauge, as you will learn later, assists you in controlling the amount of pressure used to ventilate the infant. If your anesthesia bag has a connecting site for a pressure gauge, the gauge *must* be attached for the bag to inflate.

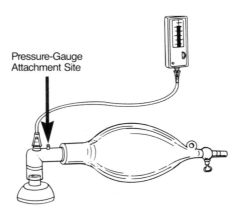

Pressure-Gauge
Attachment Site

Practice

Check to see whether your bag has a site for connecting a pressure gauge. If so, attach a gauge to the bag.

How the Bag Works

To provide you with an understanding of how an anesthesia bag works, the following topics will be discussed:
- Inflating the bag,
- Maintaining appropriate inflation, and
- Using oxygen with the bag.

Inflating the Bag

The anesthesia bag requires a compressed gas source for inflation. When the gas flows into the bag, under ordinary circumstances it will continue through the patient outlet without inflating the bag. In order to make the bag inflate, you need to keep the oxygen from escaping. You can do this by blocking the patient outlet so that the gas is trapped in the bag. In actual practice, this is done when the face mask is applied to the infant's face.

Thus, the fundamental principle upon which the inflation of an anesthesia bag depends is placing the mask over an infant's face. This "blocks" the outlet and allows the bag to inflate. You can see that when an infant is being resuscitated, the bag will not fill unless the mask is tightly sealed over the infant's mouth and nose.

Since the inflation of the bag depends on a sealed system, the bag will not inflate if:

- The mask is not properly sealed,

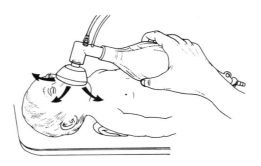

- There is a tear in the bag,

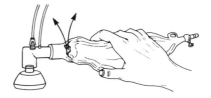

• The flow-control valve is open too far,

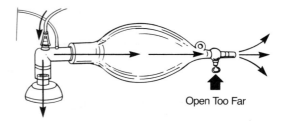

Open Too Far

• The pressure gauge is missing.

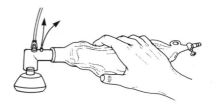

Practice

Turn the flowmeter on to 5–8 liters/minute. Note that the bag does not inflate fully. Now block the patient outlet with your thumb or hand and note that the bag expands.

Maintaining Appropriate Inflation

There are two ways you can adjust the amount of air/oxygen in most anesthesia bags:
• By adjusting the flowmeter, you regulate how much air/oxygen *enters* the bag.
• By adjusting the flow-control valve (if your bag has one), you regulate how much air/oxygen *escapes from* the bag.

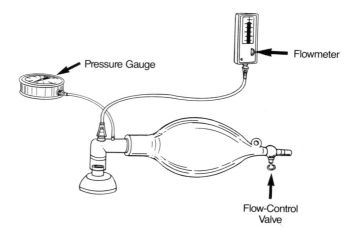

Pressure Gauge

Flowmeter

Flow-Control Valve

The flowmeter and flow-control valve should be set so that the bag is inflated to the point where it is comfortable to manage and does not completely deflate with each ventilation. An overinflated bag is difficult to manage. With practice, you will be able to make the necessary adjustments to achieve this balance.

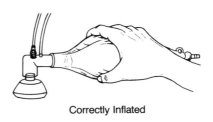

Correctly Inflated

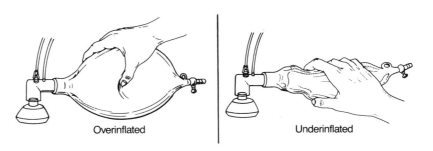

Overinflated   Underinflated

Note:

If your bag does not have a flow-control valve, you must carefully adjust the flowmeter to maintain a half-filled bag.

Practice

Close the flow-control valve of your resuscitation bag halfway.

Turn the flowmeter to 5–8 liters/minute, then block the patient outlet with your thumb (or hand). Observe the bag expanding.

Take your thumb off the patient outlet and let the bag deflate.

Increase the flow of oxygen to 10–12 liters/minute, and again block the patient outlet with your thumb. Note that the bag now fills more rapidly.

Next, observe the effect that changing the flow-control valve has on how quickly the bag inflates. Let the bag deflate, and turn the flowmeter back to 5–8 liters/minute. With the patient outlet blocked, observe what happens to the bag when you open and close the flow-control valve.

Using Oxygen With the Bag

When using an anesthesia bag, you inflate the bag with compressed oxygen. Once the oxygen enters the bag, it is not diluted, as it is in a self-inflating bag (as you will learn later). Thus, whatever concentration of oxygen you put into the bag is the *same* concentration that is delivered to the patient. Therefore, if the tubing from the bag is connected to a source of 100% oxygen, either from a wall outlet or tank, 100% oxygen will be delivered to the baby.

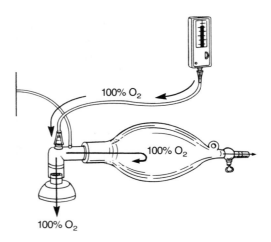

If you want to provide less than 100% oxygen, you need to use an oxygen blender. A blender is a piece of equipment that mixes or "blends" varying amounts of compressed air and oxygen. By merely turning a dial on the blender, you can obtain any desired concentration of oxygen, from 21% to 100%. For example, a blender set at 60% will provide 60% oxygen. If using an anesthesia bag, the patient would receive 60% oxygen.

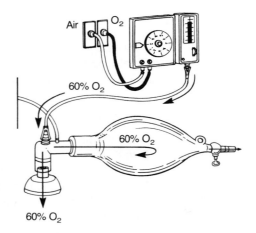

Free-flow Oxygen Via Anesthesia Bag

An anesthesia bag and mask can be used to deliver free-flow oxygen. The mask should be loosely applied to the face, allowing some gas to escape around the edges. If the mask is held tightly to the face, pressure can build up in the bag and be transmitted to the infant's lungs.

The anesthesia bag should not inflate when used to provide free-flow oxygen because pressure will not build up in the bag.

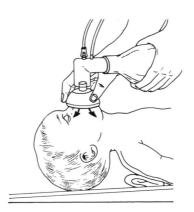

Practice

This practice exercise deals with the parts of an anesthesia bag and with filling the bag. Use your anesthesia bag as you go through the exercise. If you have any problems in completing the exercise or you are uncomfortable in doing it, talk with your instructor or supervisor.

You should have an anesthesia bag, oxygen tubing, a flowmeter, and, if applicable, a pressure gauge.

- On the bag, identify:
  - The oxygen inlet
  - The patient outlet—where the mask and ET tube attach
  - The flow-control valve
  - The pressure-gauge attachment site
- Attach the oxygen tubing to the bag
- Be sure the pressure gauge is attached
- Practice inflating the bag by turning on the flowmeter while blocking the patient outlet/mask with your hand.

Practice Activity 1

You will need to complete this practice activity *only* if you use anesthesia bags in your hospital. (However, you may complete it even if you do not use anesthesia bags.)

Fill In

Fill in the appropriate answer for each blank.
Using the drawing below, identify the two parts of an anesthesia bag:

1. _____ Gas inlet

2. _____ Patient outlet

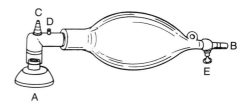

3. By adjusting the _____, you regulate how much air/oxygen *enters* an anesthesia bag.

4. By adjusting the _____, you regulate how much air/oxygen *escapes from* the bag.

5. If an anesthesia bag is connected to a 100% oxygen source, _____% oxygen will be delivered to the baby.

6. An oxygen blender used with an anesthesia bag and set at 80% will deliver _____% oxygen to the patient.

True/False

Place a **T** in front of each statement that is **true** and an **F** in front of each **false** one.

7. _____ An anesthesia bag will not inflate unless the patient outlet is blocked.

8. _____ If your anesthesia bag doesn't have a flow-control valve, you must carefully adjust the flowmeter to maintain a properly filled bag.

9. _____ After oxygen enters an anesthesia bag, it is diluted with room air.

10. _____ If you want less than 100% oxygen when using an anesthesia bag, you need to use an oxygen blender.

Fill In

11. _____ Select the picture that illustrates correct inflation of an anesthesia bag.

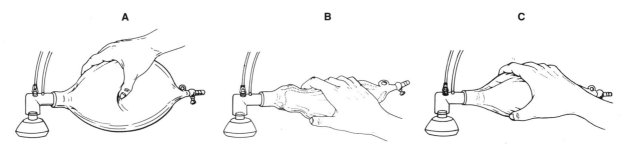

A   B   C

Multiple Choice

12–15. In the following list, place an "X" in front of each factor that might prevent an anesthesia bag from inflating.

_____ **A.** A tear in the bag

_____ **B.** Flow-control valve closed

_____ **C.** Flow-control valve completely open

_____ **D.** A leak between the mask and the infant's face

_____ **E.** Pressure gauge not attached to gauge connector

Matching

Match the parts of an anesthesia bag (listed at the right) with the descriptions given at the left.

Descriptions

16. _____ The part of an anesthesia bag where air exits from the bag to the patient.

17. _____ The part of the bag where compressed gas enters the bag.

18. _____ The part that permits air to escape.

Parts

A. Gas inlet

B. Flow-control valve

C. Patient outlet

Practice Activity 1: Answers

Carefully check your answers against the ones given below. Then review the text material for any items where you had trouble.

Fill In

1. Gas inlet — **C**

2. Patient outlet — **A**

3. Flowmeter

4. Flow-control valve

5. 100%

6. 80%

True/False

7. True

8. True

9. False — It is *not* diluted once it is in the bag. Thus, the concentration of oxygen that goes into the bag is the same concentration that is delivered to the patient.

10. True

Fill In

11. C

Multiple Choice

12–15. <u>X</u> **A.** A tear in the bag

<u>X</u> **C.** Flow-control valve completely open

<u>X</u> **D.** A leak between the mask and the infant's face

<u>X</u> **E.** Pressure gauge not attached to gauge connector

Matching

16. C

17. A

18. B

Decision

If . . .	Then . . .
You were correct on at least 17 of the 18 items . . .	Very good! You are ready to go on. Proceed to the next section if you also use self-inflating bags. Otherwise, turn to page 3A-27.
You had more than 1 incorrect answer . . .	Review the information related to the items you missed, then try again to answer those questions. When you have mastered the entire practice activity, go ahead.

Self-Inflating Bag

If you use a self-inflating resuscitation bag, study this section carefully.

Inflation of Bag

The self-inflating bag is designed so that it inflates automatically as you release your grip on the bag. It does not require a compressed gas source in order to fill.

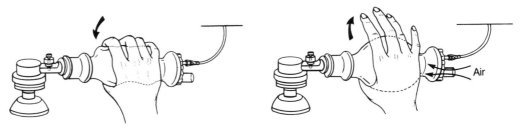

Parts

There are four parts of the self-inflating bag you should be able to identify:
- Air inlet
- Oxygen inlet
- Patient outlet
- Valve assembly

Air Inlet

As the bag reexpands following compression, air is drawn into the bag through a one-way valve that may be located at either end of the bag, depending on the design of the bag. This valve is called the *air inlet*.

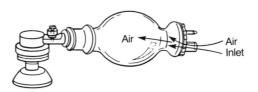

Practice

Look at the bag or bags in front of you and locate the air inlet. In most bags, the air inlet is the largest opening. You may need to squeeze the bag several times to identify where air enters the bag.

Oxygen Inlet

Every self-inflating bag has an *oxygen inlet,* which is usually located near the air inlet. The oxygen inlet is a small nipple or projection to which oxygen tubing can be attached when oxygen is needed. In the self-inflating bag, an oxygen tube does *not* need to be attached in order for the bag to function. It *does* need to be attached if the infant is to be resuscitated with an oxygen-enriched air mixture rather than with room air.

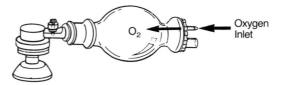

Practice

Identify where the oxygen tube connects to your resuscitation bag. Practice attaching the oxygen tube to this inlet.

Patient Outlet

The *patient outlet* is where air exits from the bag to the infant and where the mask and ET tube attach.

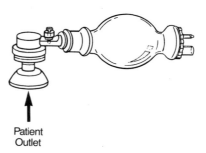

Practice

Find the patient outlet on your bag, so you will know where to attach a mask or ET tube.

Valve Assembly

Self-inflating bags have a *valve assembly* positioned between the bag and the patient outlet.

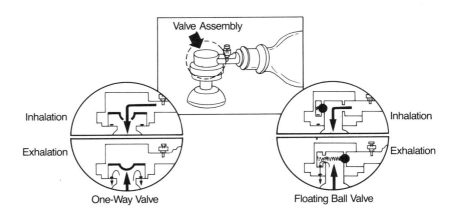

When the bag is squeezed during ventilation, the valve opens, releasing oxygen/air to the patient. When the bag reinflates (during the exhalation phase of the cycle), the valve is closed. This prevents the patient's exhaled air from entering the bag and being rebreathed. You should become familiar with the valve assembly—what it looks like and how it responds as you squeeze and release the bag. If it is missing or malfunctioning, the bag should not be used.

Practice

Identify the valve assembly on your bag. Squeeze and release the bag several times, observing how the valve moves as it opens and closes.

Note:

In many self-inflating bags, due to the valve assembly, oxygen flows from the bag only while the bag is being compressed. Since oxygen flow is not continuous, these bags *cannot* be used to provide free-flow oxygen.

Optional Part

Pressure-Gauge Attachment Site

Some self-inflating bags have a site for attaching a pressure gauge. The pressure gauge attachment site usually consists of a small hole or projection close to the patient outlet. If your bag has such a site, the gauge must be attached or air will leak through the opening, preventing adequate pressures from being generated.

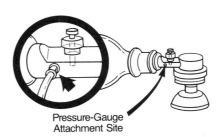

Pressure-Gauge
Attachment Site

Practice

Check to see if your bag has a special site for connecting a pressure gauge. If so, attach a gauge to the bag.

Using the Bag With Oxygen

All babies requiring positive-pressure ventilation at birth should be ventilated with a high concentration of oxygen (90–100%). Because oxygen is considered to be a drug and its use in neonates must be carefully controlled, it is important that you know the approximate concentration (%) of oxygen being administered to an infant during resuscitation.

Remember that oxygen can be brought into a self-inflating bag through tubing connected to an oxygen source. Each time the bag reinflates after you squeeze it, however, *room air* is drawn into the bag by way of the air inlet. The room air dilutes the concentration of oxygen in the bag. This means that even though you have 100% oxygen flowing through the O_2 inlet, it is diluted by the room air that enters each time the bag reinflates. As a result, the concentration of oxygen actually received by the patient is greatly reduced—it is somewhere in the range of 40%.

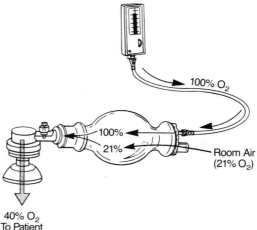

100% O_2

100%

21%

Room Air (21% O_2)

40% O_2
To Patient

This low concentration of oxygen (40%) is inadequate for ventilating an infant at birth—a time when a high concentration of oxygen (90–100%) should be used.

Oxygen Reservoir

High concentrations of oxygen can be achieved with a self-inflating bag through the use of both the oxygen tubing and an *oxygen reservoir.* An oxygen reservoir is an appliance that can be placed over the bag's air inlet. This reservoir provides a chamber filled with a high concentration of oxygen and prevents the majority of room air from entering the bag and mixing with the oxygen. This permits administration of as high as 90–100% oxygen with a self-inflating bag.

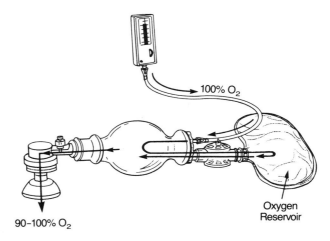

100% O₂

Oxygen
Reservoir

90–100% O₂

There are several different types of oxygen reservoirs, but they all perform the same function.

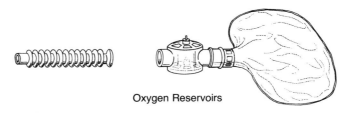

Oxygen Reservoirs

Many of the oxygen reservoirs are not completely sealed units; therefore, a very small amount of room air can enter the bag during reinflation. For this reason, the concentration of oxygen provided by this method may not be 100%, but somewhere between 90% and 100%.

As you have learned, high concentrations of oxygen are essential for resuscitation of infants at birth. You also learned that self-inflating bags without an oxygen reservoir may deliver only 40% oxygen, which is not sufficient for neonatal resuscitation. This means that *self-inflating bags without oxygen reservoirs are totally inadequate* for resuscitation in the delivery room. Therefore, all *self-inflating bags used in a delivery room must have oxygen reservoirs attached so that the bags are capable of delivering a high concentration of oxygen.*

Practice

For practice, prepare your self-inflating bag to provide 90–100% oxygen. Attach an oxygen tube to the oxygen inlet and an oxygen reservoir to the air inlet. The other end of the oxygen tubing should be connected to an oxygen flowmeter or a blender set at 100%.

If you do not understand the purpose of the oxygen reservoir or how it works to increase the oxygen concentration in the bag, ask someone to help you.

Practice Activity 2

You will need to take this practice activity only if you use *self-inflating bags* where you work. (You are welcome to take it even if you do not use self-inflating bags.)

Fill In

Write in the appropriate answer to fill each blank.
Use the drawing to identify the following parts of a self-inflating bag:

1. _____ Air inlet

2. _____ Oxygen inlet

3. _____ Patient outlet

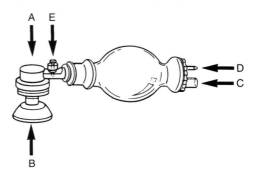

4. All self-inflating bags used in the resuscitation of a newborn infant must have a (an) _____ attached in order to provide a high concentration of oxygen.

5. When a self-inflating bag without an oxygen reservoir is connected to an oxygen source, what is the approximate concentration of oxygen actually received by the patient? _____%

6. When an oxygen reservoir is used with a self-inflating bag, what is the concentration of oxygen that can be achieved? _____ to _____%

Matching

Match the parts of a self-inflating bag (given in the right-hand column) with the descriptions given at the left.

Descriptions

7. _____ A small nipple to which oxygen tubing can be attached.

8. _____ A one-way valve through which air is drawn into the bag as the bag reexpands following compression.

9. _____ Opens and closes during assisted ventilation, providing the infant with fresh oxygen/air and preventing rebreathing of exhaled air.

10. _____ Where the air exits from the bag to the infant (also, where the bag and ET tube attach).

11. _____ An appliance that can be placed over the resuscitation bag's air inlet.

Parts

A. Air inlet

B. Oxygen inlet

C. Oxygen reservoir

D. Patient outlet

E. Valve assembly

True/False

Place a **T** in front of each **true** statement and an **F** in front of each one that is **false.**

12. _____ The self-inflating bag must be connected to a compressed gas source before it will fill.

13. _____ The self-inflating bag is a truly portable resuscitation bag.

14. _____ In the self-inflating bag, an oxygen tube needs to be attached if the infant is to be resuscitated with an oxygen-enriched air mixture.

15. _____ When oxygen is used with a self-inflating bag, the air inlet remains closed when the bag reinflates.

16. _____ High concentrations of oxygen, 90–100%, can be achieved with a self-inflating bag if an oxygen reservoir is used.

17. _____ All oxygen reservoirs are sealed units that do not permit any room air to enter the bag during reinflation.

18. _____ Self-inflating bags without oxygen reservoirs should not be used for resuscitation in the delivery room.

Practice

This practice exercise wil help you review certain important concepts and skills in using a self-inflating bag.

You should have in front of you one of each type of self-inflating bag you will be using. Also, you should have some oxygen tubing and an oxygen reservoir.

On the bag identify:

• The oxygen inlet,
• The air inlet,
• The patient outlet,
• The valve assembly, and
• A place to connect a pressure gauge, if there is one.

Prepare the bag to deliver high concentrations of oxygen by attaching:

• The oxygen tubing, and
• The oxygen reservoir.

Practice Activity 2: Answers

Carefully check your responses against the answers given here. Be sure to review the information related to any items about which you are uncertain.

Fill In

1. **C**—Air inlet

2. **D**—Oxygen inlet

3. **B**—Patient outlet

4. Oxygen reservoir

5. 40%

6. 90–100%

Matching

7. **B**

8. **A**

9. **E**

10. **D**

11. **C**

True/False

12. **False**—The self-inflating bag automatically inflates when you release your grip on the bag. It does not need a compressed gas source.

13. **True**

14. **True**

15. **False**—The air inlet opens during reinflation regardless of whether oxygen is flowing into the bag. If no oxygen reservoir is used, this allows room air to enter the bag, reducing the concentration of oxygen received by the patient.

16. **True**

17. **False**—They are not completely sealed, so a very small amount of room air can enter the bag. This is why the concentration of oxygen provided is stated as a range of 90–100%, rather than 100%.

18. **True**

Decision

If . . .	Then . . .
Your score was 17 or more . . .	You have done well on this practice activity. Go on to the next section.
You missed more than 1 . . .	Carefully go back over the information the lesson gave for the items you missed. When you have the correct information well in mind, go ahead.

Safety Features

Now that you have learned the basics of how a resuscitation bag works, let's take a look at two safety features that are built into bags to help control the amount of pressure that goes into the lungs. These safety mechanisms help prevent overinflation of the infant's lungs, which could result in rupture of the alveoli, producing a pneumothorax. These safety features are the:

• Pressure-release valve and

• Pressure gauge.

Any resuscitation bag used for neonates, regardless of whether it is an anesthesia bag or self-inflating bag, should have at least *one* of these two features.

Pressure-Release Valve

Self-inflating bag

A pressure-release valve, more commonly called a *pop-off valve*, is a feature found on many resuscitation bags, especially self-inflating bags.

Pressure-release valves are generally set to release at 30–35 cm H_2O on self-inflating bags. Therefore, if pressures greater than 30–35 cm are generated, the valve opens, preventing pressure from being transmitted to the infant.

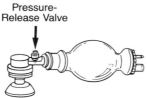

Pressure-
Release Valve

In some self-inflating bags, the pop-off valve can be temporarily occluded or bypassed to allow pressures greater than 35 cm H_2O to be administered. This may occasionally be necessary to effectively ventilate a neonate's nonaerated lungs, especially with the first few breaths. Extreme care must be taken not to use excessive pressure during the few ventilations in which the pop-off valve is bypassed. A pressure gauge should be attached to any self-inflating bag in which the pop-off valve can be bypassed.

Anesthesia bag

Some anesthesia bags contain an adjustable pop-off valve that can usually be found in the elbow between the bag and the mask. This valve may be adjusted to release at a desired pressure.

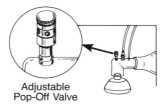

Adjustable
Pop-Off Valve

It will be impossible for you to know the exact pressure you are delivering if your bag is equipped with only a pressure-release valve and no pressure gauge. If the pressure-release valve is adjustable, you must have a pressure gauge to know the pressure at which the pop-off valve is set.

Practice

Check the self-inflating bag you are using to see whether it has a pressure-release valve. You may need to ask someone to point it out. Usually, however, you can locate it by blocking the patient outlet and squeezing the bag with considerable force. The pressure-release valve will be a small opening that releases air when excessive pressure is applied to the bag. When this happens, you usually hear a change in the sound and may actually be able to see the valve open.

Because you cannot produce exact pressure (without the use of a pressure gauge), you should practice squeezing the bag (with the patient outlet blocked), using a pressure somewhat less than that needed to actuate the pressure-release valve. This will give you a feel for pressures of 25–30 cm H_2O.

Now, once again give the bag a hard squeeze and listen for the change in sound. When you hear the change, you will know that you have exerted pressure of more than 35 cm H_2O and the extra pressure has escaped through the pressure-release valve.

Pressure Gauge

A pressure gauge is an extra piece of equipment attached to the bag by means of a small tube, at a point close to the patient outlet. It measures the pressure generated by the bag in centimeters (cm) of water. This gauge allows the person using the bag to more precisely control the pressure of the air or oxygen being delivered to the patient.

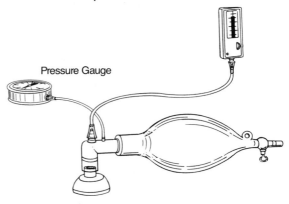

Pressure Gauge

Pressure Gauge With Pressure Release Valve

Some pressure gauges also come with a pressure release valve. The valve can be set to go off at a desired pressure.

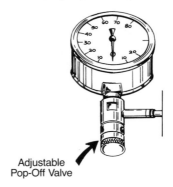

Adjustable
Pop-Off Valve

Practice

If your bag is fitted with a pressure gauge, practice delivering specific ventilation pressures. For the gauge to register, you will need to hold your hand tightly over the mask or patient outlet as you squeeze the bag.

Practice delivering the following pressures, which are pressures used in ventilating newborns.

- 15–20 cm H_2O
- 20–30 cm H_2O
- 30–40 cm H_2O

You will find that you do not have to squeeze the bag very hard in order to get a reading on the gauge. It is very important that you learn how to control the pressure used in ventilating the patient. You will learn more about specific pressures later, in Part B of this lesson.

Resuscitation Masks

Introduction

Now that you have had an opportunity to become familiar with the resuscitation bags, let's consider the masks you will use with the bags. Masks come in a variety of shapes, sizes, and materials. The selection of a specific mask for use with a particular infant will depend on how well the mask fits the infant's face and how easy it is to use in obtaining a seal. In this portion of the lesson you will learn the differences in the types of rims and shapes of masks, as well as the criteria for selecting a mask of the proper size.

Rim

Noncushioned

Cushioned

Resuscitation masks have rims that are either *cushioned* or *noncushioned*.

Some masks are constructed *without* a padded, soft rim. Such a mask usually has a very firm, abrupt edge to the rim. One must be careful in using such a mask because the *noncushioned* rim can cause several problems:

- Because it does not easily conform to the shape of the baby's face, it requires greater pressure to form a seal than does a cushioned mask.
- It can damage the eyes if the mask is improperly positioned.
- It can bruise the neonate's face if the mask is applied too firmly.

The soft rim on a cushioned mask is made from either a soft, flexible material, such as foam rubber, or an air-inflated ring. A cushioned-rim mask has several advantages over a mask without a cushioned rim:

- The rim conforms more easily to the shape of the infant's face, making it easier to form a seal.
- It requires less pressure on the infant's face to obtain a seal.
- There is less chance of damaging the infant's eyes if the mask is incorrectly positioned.

Practice

Check to see whether the masks you are using are cushioned. If they are, look to see if they have a plug or valve that can be used to reinflate the rim, should it deflate. If so, practice deflating and reinflating the rim.

Shape

Masks come in two shapes.

Round	Anatomically Shaped
	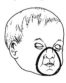

Round

A round mask can be effective in obtaining a seal for ventilation but can also present some problems. If the correct size is not selected, a seal cannot be formed, for it may not fit over the mouth and nose correctly. Additionally, if the mask is too large, pressure may be exerted on the eyes and can cause damage.

Anatomically Shaped

Some masks are shaped to fit the contours of the face. These masks are referred to as *anatomically shaped* masks. They are made to be placed on the face in a particular direction with the most pointed part of the mask fitting over the nose.

You will find it easier to obtain a seal with an anatomical mask. Also, there is less chance of causing damage to the eyes because the rim is contoured to fit between the eyes and nose.

Practice

If you are using an anatomically shaped mask, determine which part is meant to fit over the nose and which part over the chin.

Size

Masks come in several sizes. Your resuscitation tray should contain masks suitable for small premature infants as well as for fullterm infants. There should be masks for infants from 2 to 10 pounds.

Fit

For the mask to be the correct size, the rim must cover the tip of the chin, the mouth, and the nose, but not the eyes.
- Too large—possible eye damage.
- Too small—will not cover the mouth and nose and may occlude the nose.

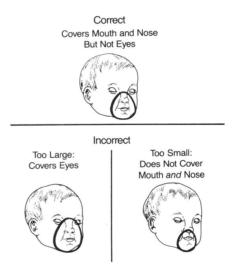

Correct
Covers Mouth and Nose
But Not Eyes

Incorrect

Too Large:
Covers Eyes

Too Small:
Does Not Cover
Mouth *and* Nose

Practice

Using the resuscitation manikin, check the masks you have. Determine which ones are too large and which ones are too small, and identify the ones that are the correct size. You can also practice selecting appropriately sized masks for infants in the nursery.

Practice Activity 3

Use the following practice activity items to test your knowledge of key ideas dealing with resuscitation masks and the safety features of resuscitation bags.

Fill In

1–2. Every resuscitation bag should have at least one of two safety features for regulating pressure. State the two features.

   • _____

   • _____

3–4. When selecting a mask, make sure that the rim covers the tip of the chin, the _____, and the _____, but does not cover the eyes.

True/False

5. _____ Pressure-release valves are generally set to release at 50–60 cm H_2O.

6. _____ If the bag you are using has no pressure gauge, you cannot judge the exact pressure you are delivering to the infant.

7. _____ Anatomically shaped masks should be positioned with the more pointed end over the chin.

8. _____ Eye damage can occur from an improperly positioned mask.

Selecting

In the following items, use an "X" to show the type of resuscitation mask to which each statement refers.

Rim	Noncushioned	Cushioned
9. Conforms more easily to shape of face; easier to form seal		
10. Requires greater pressure to form seal		
11. Can bruise infant's face if applied too firmly		
12. Requires less pressure to obtain seal		

Practice Activity 3: Answers

The answers given below should be carefully checked against your own responses.

Fill In

1–2. Pressure-release valve (pop-off valve)

Pressure gauge

3–4. Mouth

Nose

True/False

5. False — They release at *30–35* cm H_2O.

6. True

7. False — The more pointed end should be over the nose.

8. True

Selecting

Rim	Noncushioned	Cushioned
9. Conforms more easily to shape of face; easier to form seal		X
10. Requires greater pressure to form seal	X	
11. Can bruise infant's face if applied too firmly	X	
12. Requires less pressure to obtain seal		X

Decision

If ...	Then ...
You had at least 11 items correct ...	Good work! Go right on to the posttest.
You had fewer than 11 correct ...	Be sure you understand the information related to each item you missed. Answer those questions again; then go ahead.

Posttest
Lesson 3A—
Use of a Resuscitation Bag and Mask: Equipment

Name _____ Date _____

This posttest is designed to let you test yourself on your understanding of resuscitation bags and masks. Follow the directions for each part.

Fill In

1–2. Every resuscitation bag should have at least one of two safety features for regulating pressure. State the two features.

- _____

- _____

3–5. When selecting a mask, make sure that the rim covers the tip of the _____, the _____, and the _____, but does not cover the eyes.

Selection

Which of the following pictures show that the mask chosen for the infant is the correct size? In the space provided, place the letter of each correct picture.

6–7. _____

A   B   C

D   E

True/False

8. _____ Pressure-release valves are generally set to release at 50–60 cm H_2O.

9. _____ Anatomically shaped masks should be positioned with the more pointed end over the chin.

10. _____ Too much pressure on the mask can bruise the face.

11. _____ A pneumothorax can result from ventilating the infant with too much pressure.

Fill In

If you use an anesthesia bag, complete Questions 12–16. If you use only the self-inflating bag, move ahead to Question 17.

12. By adjusting the _____, you regulate how much air/oxygen *enters* an anesthesia bag.

13. By adjusting the _____, you regulate how much air/oxygen *escapes from* the bag.

14. If the tubing from an anesthesia bag is connected to 100% oxygen, _____% oxygen will be delivered to the baby.

15. An oxygen blender used with an anesthesia bag and set at 45% will deliver _____% oxygen to the patient.

16. What problem will occur in using an anesthesia bag, if any of the following are present: a tear in the bag, a fully open flow-control valve, no pressure gauge attached to the connector site, a leak between the mask and face?

_____

If you use a self-inflating bag, complete the following questions. If you only use an anesthesia bag, you are finished with the posttest and do not need to complete the remaining questions.

True/False

Place a **T** in front of each **true** statement and an **F** in front of each one that is **false.**

17. _____ The self-inflating bag must be connected to oxygen before it will fill.

18. _____ In the self-inflating bag, an oxygen tube needs to be attached if the infant is to be resuscitated with an oxygen-enriched air mixture.

19. _____ A self-inflating bag with a connection site for a pressure gauge does not need to have the gauge connected for the bag to work properly.

20. _____ Self-inflating bags with valves that only open when the bag is being compressed should not be used to deliver free-flow oxygen.

Fill In

21. All self-inflating bags used in the resuscitation of an infant at birth must have a (an) _____ attached in order to provide a high concentration of oxygen.

22. When a self-inflating bag without an oxygen reservoir is connected to an oxygen source, what is the approximate concentration of oxygen actually received by the patient? _____%

23. When an oxygen reservoir is used with a self-inflating bag, what is the concentration of oxygen that can be achieved? _____ to _____%

Lesson 3A Posttest: Answers

Check your answers with those given here.

Fill In

1–2. Pressure-release valve (pop-off valve)

Pressure gauge

3–5. Tip of the *chin,* the *mouth,* and the *nose.*

Selection

6–7. B and **C**

True/False

8. False—They release at *30–35* cm H_2O.

9. False—The more pointed end should be over the nose.

10. True

11. True

Anesthesia Bag:

Fill In

12. Flowmeter

13. Flow-control valve

14. 100%

15. 45%

16. The bag will not inflate—or at least not inflate properly

---

Self-Inflating Bag:

True/False

17. False—The self-inflating bag automatically inflates when you release your grip on it. It does not need a compressed gas source.

18. True

19. False—If the gauge is not attached, air will leak through the opening, preventing adequate pressure from being generated.

20. True

Fill-In

21. Oxygen reservoir

22. 40%

23. 90-100%

Decision

If . . .	Then . . .
You answered all 23 questions and had at least 21 correct . . .	Good! You have successfully completed the posttest.
or	
You omitted questions related to the anesthesia bag *or* the self-inflating bag and missed no more than 2 items . . .	
You missed more than 2 items . . .	You should review the information related to those you missed, and then take the posttest again.

Use of a Resuscitation Bag and Mask: Ventilating the Infant

Lesson 3B

Contents

Use of a Resuscitation Bag and Mask: Ventilating the Infant

Lesson 3B

Overview of Lesson 3B

In Lesson 3A, you became thoroughly familiar with the resuscitation bags and masks you will be using. Now you will learn how to actually use this equipment to ventilate an infant. Lesson 3C will deal with how to incorporate ventilation into the entire resuscitation procedure.

In this lesson you will first learn how to prepare and check the bag and mask to be sure they function properly.

Second, you will learn the hardest part of ventilating an infant, obtaining an airtight seal between the face and mask.

Next, you will learn how rapidly to ventilate an infant and how to determine the amount of pressure to use.

Last, you will become acquainted with additional equipment occasionally used with the bag and mask: an oral airway, an 8 Fr. feeding tube, and syringe used to remove air and secretions from the stomach.

Objectives

Knowledge

When you have finished this lesson you should be able to:

- Identify the maximum size resuscitation bag that should be used in neonates.
- State the oxygen concentration that should be used when ventilating an infant at birth.
- State the correct rate for ventilating a newborn.
- State the correct pressures to use when ventilating infants who have not taken the first breath, those with normal, healthy lungs, and those with pulmonary disease.
- State how you can determine if an infant is being properly ventilated.
- List three basic problems that can prevent lung inflation during bag-and-mask ventilation.
- When an initial attempt at bag-and-mask ventilation fails to produce observable chest expansion, list in the appropriate sequence the five steps that can be taken in an attempt to remedy the situation.
- Identify three situations when an oral airway may be required during ventilation.
- State two reasons for inserting an orogastric tube during positive-pressure ventilation, and state when the tube should be inserted.

Performance

You should also be able to:
- Select, prepare, and check a resuscitation bag and mask for use on an infant in the delivery room.
- Select the correct mask size.
- Using an infant resuscitation manikin, obtain a seal between the face and mask, and ventilate the manikin, using an appropriate rate and pressure.
- Demonstrate proper use of an orogastric catheter during bag-and-mask ventilation.

3B-3

Decision Table

If . . .	Then . . .
You feel you can pass a test on the objectives . . .	Turn to the posttest.
You wish to know more before trying the posttest . . .	Go on to the next page and begin the lesson.

Equipment Required

As you work through this lesson, you will need all of the equipment you gathered for Lesson 3A.

The resuscitation manikin, which was optional in Part A, is now mandatory. The only way to practice attaining a seal and using the appropriate pressures is to use an infant resuscitation manikin. It is important that the procedure be practiced on a *manikin* and *NEVER on a live infant*.

Additional equipment needed includes:
Clock or watch with second hand
8 Fr. feeding tube
20-cc (or larger) syringe
Infant oral airways
Adhesive tape — 1/2" x 2"
Towel or roll for placement under the shoulders (optional)

Preparing and Checking Equipment

The first step in ventilating an infant is to be certain that the bag and mask are correctly assembled and functioning. This entails:
- Selecting the proper equipment,
- Assembling it correctly, and
- Testing it for function.

Selecting Equipment

The equipment should be specifically designed for newborns. Consideration should be given to:
- Size of bag
- Oxygen capability
- Safety features
- Size of mask

Resuscitation Bag

Size

Bags used for newborn infants should not exceed 750 mL. Term neonates only require 20–30 mL with each ventilation (6–8 mL/kg). Bags larger than 750 mL make it difficult to provide such small volumes. Some self-inflating bags have a capacity as small as 240 mL.

Oxygen Capability

Infants who require positive-pressure ventilation *at birth,* should be initially ventilated with a high concentration of oxygen (90–100%). This can be accomplished with either:
- An anesthesia bag, or
- A self-inflating bag with an oxygen reservoir.

Safety Features

To minimize complications resulting from high airway pressures, the bag should have either a:
- Pressure-release valve, or
- Pressure gauge.

Oxygen Source

In order to provide a high concentration of oxygen, a source of 100% oxygen is required along with oxygen tubing and a flowmeter.

Mask

A mask of the proper size should be selected. It should cover the chin, mouth, and nose.

Assembling Equipment

The bag should be assembled and connected to oxygen so that it will provide the necessary 90–100%. If a self-inflating bag is used, be sure the oxygen reservoir is attached. Last, connect the mask to the bag.

Testing Equipment

Once the equipment has been selected and assembled, check the bag and mask to be sure they function properly. Optimal success in using a bag and mask requires more than up-to-date equipment and a skilled operator—the equipment must be in working order. Bags that have cracks or tears, valves that stick or leak, or masks that are cracked or deflated must not be used. The equipment should be checked prior to each delivery. The operator should check it again just prior to its use.

Since there are different things to check on an anesthesia bag than on a self-inflating bag, each type of bag will be discussed separately. If you do not use both types, you will only need to read about the type you are using.

Anesthesia Bag

To check an anesthesia bag, attach it to an oxygen source so that it will inflate. Adjust the flowmeter to 5–8 liters, which provides a flow of oxygen that allows the bag to be at least three-quarters full but not tense. If you have a flow-control valve, make sure you have adjusted that if necessary. Block the patient outlet in order to make sure the bag fills properly. Do this by making an airtight seal between the patient outlet or mask and the palm of your hand.

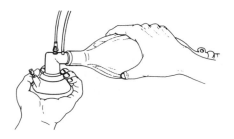

Does the bag fill properly?

If not:

- Is there a crack or tear in the bag?
- Is the flow-control valve open all the way?
- Is the pressure gauge missing?
- Is the patient outlet *completely* blocked?

If the bag fills, squeeze the bag:

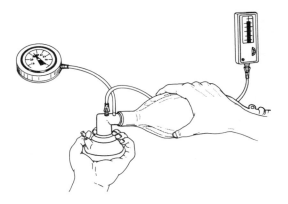

- Do you feel pressure against your hand?
- Does the pressure gauge register 30–40 cm H_2O pressure?

If the bag does not fill properly or does not generate adequate pressure, obtain another bag and begin again.

Self-Inflating Bag

To check a self-inflating bag, block the mask or patient outlet by making an *airtight* seal with the palm of your hand. Then squeeze the bag:

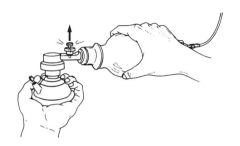

- Do you feel pressure against your hand?
- Does the pressure gauge register 30–40 cm H_2O pressure?
- Can you force the pressure-release valve open?
- Is the valve assembly present and moving as it should?

If not:
- Is there a crack or leak in the bag?
- Is the pressure gauge missing?
- Is the pressure-release valve missing or stuck closed?
- Is the patient outlet *completely* blocked?

If your bag generates adequate pressure and the safety features are working, while the mask/patient outlet is blocked, check to see:
- Does the bag reinflate quickly when you release your grip?

If there is any problem with the bag, obtain a new one. Self-inflating bags usually have more parts than an anesthesia bag. With cleaning, parts may be left out, assembled incorrectly, or left moist, causing them to "stick."

You should become very familiar with the type of bag you are using. You must know exactly how to check it to quickly determine whether it is functioning properly.

Mask

Check the mask carefully for any cracks or defects in the rim.

Practice

To become more familiar with checking your equipment, go around your unit and test each bag and mask. Are they all functional? Be sure you handle the equipment with clean hands, so as not to contaminate it.

Practice Activity 1

Use this practice activity to test your knowledge of the key concepts and principles of preparing and checking the equipment used in ventilating an infant.

Multiple Choice

1. Resuscitation bags for neonates should not exceed:

    _____ **A.** 240 mL

    _____ **B.** 500 mL

    _____ **C.** 750 mL

    _____ **D.** 1 liter (1000 mL)

2. With each ventilation, the fullterm neonate requires approximately:

    _____ **A.** 10–15 mL

    _____ **B.** 20–30 mL

    _____ **C.** 40–50 mL

    _____ **D.** 50–60 mL

3. Resuscitation equipment should always be checked:

    _____ **A.** Prior to each delivery

    _____ **B.** Daily

    _____ **C.** Weekly

    _____ **D.** Monthly

Fill In

4. What concentration of oxygen should be used when ventilating an infant at birth?

    _____ to _____%

Performance Activity

5. Assemble your resuscitation bag for use with a 1500 gm (3 lb. 5 oz.), premature infant.

6. Test your bag and mask to be sure they are functioning properly.

Practice Activity 1: Answers

Check your answers with those given here.

Multiple Choice

1. C

2. B

3. A

Fill In

4. 90–100%

Performance Activity

5. *Assembling the bag*
   - Did you connect an oxygen tube to the O_2 inlet on the bag and to a flowmeter or blender?
   - If using a self-inflating bag, did you attach an oxygen reservoir?
   - Did you attach a mask suitable for a 1500 gm (3 lb. 5 oz.) infant?

6. *Testing Bag and Mask*
   Anesthesia bag
   - Did you check to see if the bag can inflate by turning the liter flow to 5–8 liters/minute and blocking the patient outlet?
   - Did you squeeze the bag to see if it generates adequate pressure and is free of leaks or tears?
   - Did you check the pressure gauge to see if it registers as you squeeze the bag?

   Self-inflating bag
   - Did you block the mask/patient outlet and squeeze the bag to see if it generates adequate pressure — being free of cracks and tears?
   - Did you check the safety features?
     - Pressure gauge — did it register as you squeezed the bag?
     - Pressure-release valve — did it open when you compressed the bag firmly?
   - Did you check the valve assembly?
     - Did you check to see if the bag reinflated quickly when you released your grip?

   Mask
   - Did you check to see that it had no cracks and the rim, if cushioned, is properly inflated?

Decision

If . . .	Then . . .
You answered all 4 questions correctly and did all of the steps in the performance activity correctly . . .	Excellent. Continue to the next section.
You missed a question or left out a step in the performance activity . . .	Review the material and/or practice until the steps become automatic.

Forming and Checking Seal

Once you are sure that the equipment is functioning properly, you are ready to ventilate the infant. The most critical step in the process is to form an airtight seal between the mask and face.

At first, you will feel awkward in handling the bag and mask. By following the steps given here and taking time to practice, you will eventually be able to quickly apply the mask and obtain an effective seal—using minimal pressure to hold the mask on the face.

Position of Infant

Before beginning ventilation, the baby's position should be checked. The neck should be slightly extended to maintain an open airway. One way to accomplish this is to place a roll under the shoulders.

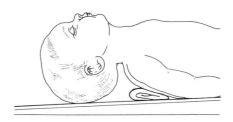

If, while caring for the infant up to this point, the baby's position has shifted, reposition before continuing.

Position of Ventilator

You will need to stand at the side or head of the infant to use the resuscitation bag effectively. This position will allow you to comfortably hold the mask on the infant's face. If you are right-handed, you will probably feel most comfortable holding the bag with your right hand and the mask with your left. If left-handed, you will probably want to control the bag with your left hand and hold the mask with your right.

It is important that the bag is positioned so that it does not block your view of the infant's chest, since you need to be able to observe the rise and fall of the chest during ventilation.

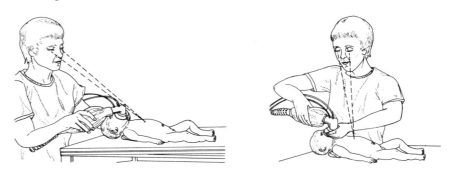

Positions With Unobstructed View of Chest

Both positions leave the chest and abdomen unobstructed for visual monitoring of the infant and for chest compressions and vascular access via the umbilical cord, should these procedures become necessary.

Positioning Mask

The mask should be applied to the face so that it covers the nose and mouth, and the edge of the chin rests within the rim of the mask. You may find it helpful to begin by cupping the chin in the mask and then covering the nose.

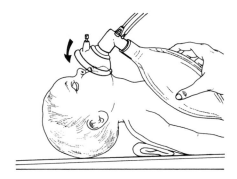

The mask is usually held on the face with the thumb and index and/or third finger encircling much of the rim of the mask, while the ring finger holds the chin in the mask.

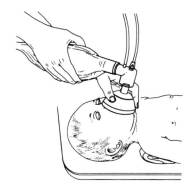

Remember, anatomically shaped masks should be positioned with the pointed end over the nose.

Once the mask is positioned, an airtight seal can be formed by using *light* downward pressure on the rim of the mask.

Caution:

Care should be taken in holding the mask. The following are "do nots":

• Do not "jam" the mask down on the face. Too much pressure can mold (flatten) the back of the head and can bruise the face.

• Do not put pressure on the throat (trachea). This could block the airway.

• Do not allow your fingers, parts of your hand, or the stem of a reinflatable cushioned rim to rest on the infant's eyes.

No Pressure on These Areas

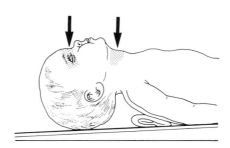

Practice

With the mask attached to the bag, use the infant manikin to practice positioning the bag and mask and forming a face/mask seal.
- Is the mask covering the tip of the chin, mouth, and nose?
- Are you using at least one finger to hold the chin to the rim of the mask?
- Are the trachea and eyes free of all pressure?
- Are you holding the bag in a comfortable position?
- Do you have an unobstructed view of the chest?

Practice the above, standing at both the head and side of the manikin.

Checking the Seal

Once the seal is formed, it is important to check that it is airtight and that the chest rises as you squeeze the bag. A moment taken at this time to make an adjustment will allow you to provide effective ventilation without delay.

The mask must be properly applied and the seal tight. Remember that the volume of the infant's lungs is only a fraction of the volume of the bag. You should never have to squeeze a bag empty to inflate the lungs of an infant.

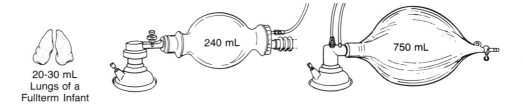

20-30 mL
Lungs of a
Fullterm Infant

240 mL

750 mL

Observing Chest Movement

Once you have positioned the mask, squeeze the bag and observe for chest movement.

A noticeable rise and fall of the chest is by far the best indication that the mask is sealed and the lungs are being inflated. The infant should appear to be taking a shallow or "easy" breath.

If the chest rises to its maximum, appearing as if the baby is taking a deep breath, the lungs are being overinflated. You are using too much pressure, and there is danger of producing a pneumothorax.

Abdominal Movement

Abdominal movement should not be used to determine whether the lungs are being properly ventilated. Abdominal movement may be due to air entering the stomach and should not be mistaken for effective ventilation.

Bilateral Breath Sounds

The presence of bilateral breath sounds indicates that the infant is being properly ventilated.

Observing for Chest Expansion

You may find that your first attempt at ventilation does not result in optimal chest expansion. If the chest expands too much, simply reduce the pressure by squeezing less firmly. However, if the chest does not expand, there could be several reasons. We will now consider some of the things you should look for in evaluating chest expansion and some of the factors that bring about inadequate chest expansion.

Inadequate Expansion

If the chest does not expand adequately, it may be for one or more of the following reasons:
- There is an inadequate seal.
- The airway is blocked.
- Not enough pressure is being given.

Inadequate Seal

If you hear or feel air escaping from around the mask, reapply the mask to the face and try to form a better seal. Use a little more pressure on the rim of the mask. *Do not* press down hard on the infant's face. The most common place for a leak to occur is between the cheek and bridge of the nose.

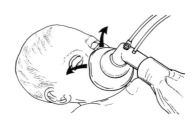

Blocked Airway

Another possible reason for insufficient ventilation of the baby's lungs is a blocked airway. To correct this:
- Check the infant's position, and extend the neck a bit farther.
- Check the mouth, oropharynx, and nose for secretions (this will not be a problem with the manikin). Suction mouth and nose if necessary.
- Try ventilating with the infant's mouth slightly open. This may be facilitated by inserting an oral airway.

Not Enough Pressure

The third possible reason for failure of the chest to rise is inadequate pressure. How you ventilate at higher pressures will depend on the equipment you are using.

- If using a bag with a *pressure gauge*, increase the pressure slightly.
- If using a bag with a *pressure-release valve,* increase the pressure until the valve actuates. If more pressure is required and it is possible to occlude the pressure-release valve, do so, and cautiously increase the pressure.

Sequence

If you don't observe chest expansion, try the following steps *in the order given* until the chest expands.

Action	Condition Corrected
1. Reapply mask to face	Inadequate seal
2. Reposition the head	Blocked airway
3. Check for secretions — suction if present	Blocked airway
4. Ventilate with infant's mouth slightly open	Blocked airway
5. Increase pressure to 20–40 cm H_2O, or until pressure-release valve is actuated (if you are using a self-inflating bag)	Not enough pressure

Practice

If you have not already done so, practice ventilating the manikin, using the steps outlined thus far in this section. Ask for assistance if you are not able to adequately form a seal and ventilate the manikin. Once you have accomplished this, you are ready to go on and learn about ventilation rate and pressures.

Practice Activity 2

Use this practice activity to test your knowledge about forming and checking an airtight seal between an infant's face and the ventilation bag.

True/False

1. _____ When skilled in using a bag and mask, you should be able to ventilate an infant, using minimal pressure to hold the mask to the face.

2. _____ During ventilation, the mask should cover the mouth, nose, and tip of the chin, but not the eyes.

3. _____ To provide an open airway when using a resuscitation bag and mask, the head should be pulled back, hyperextending the neck.

4. _____ Too much pressure on the mask can mold the back of the infant's head and can bruise the face.

5. _____ Chest expansion indicates that you have an adequate mask/face seal.

6. _____ Abdominal movement is a good indicator that the lungs are being properly ventilated.

Completion

7. Briefly describe the main consideration in positioning a resuscitation bag as you ventilate an infant.

_____

_____

8. When ventilating an infant, you should be careful that your fingers or parts of your hand are not applying pressure to what two areas?

   • _____

   • _____

9–11. You ventilate an infant two to three times to check the seal, but you notice that the chest does not rise. What three basic problems should you consider as being possibly responsible for the lack of chest movement?

   • _____

   • _____

   • _____

If you do not observe chest expansion, you should quickly remedy the situation so you can ventilate the baby. List, in order, the five steps you would go through to correct the problem.

12. _____

13. _____

14. _____

15. _____

16. _____

Multiple Choice

17. Which of the following are true of an infant being properly ventilated? Place an "X" in front of each that applies.

_____ **A.** You will see good chest expansion—the infant will appear to be taking a deep breath.

_____ **B.** The pressure gauge will register the appropriate ventilation pressure for the particular infant, although you may not see a rise and fall of the chest.

_____ **C.** You will see chest movement—the infant will appear to be taking a shallow or "easy" breath.

Practice Activity 2: Answers

Check your answer with those given here.

True/False

1. **True**

2. **True**

3. **False** — The position should be the same as you learned previously — with the neck *slightly* extended. Hyperextending the neck decreases air entry.

4. **True**

5. **True**

6. **False** — Abdominal movement may be due to air entering the stomach and should not be mistaken for effective ventilation.

Completion

7. The resuscitation bag should be positioned so you have an *unobstructed view of the chest.*

8. • The eyes
   • The throat (or trachea)

9–11. • Inadequate seal
   • Blocked airway
   • Not enough pressure

12. Reapply mask to face

13. Reposition the head

14. Check for secretions — suction if necessary

15. Ventilate with infant's mouth slightly open

16. Increase pressure

Multiple Choice

17. **X C.** You will see chest movement — the infant will appear to be taking a shallow or "easy" breath.
   (If you answered **B,** remember that the pressure gauge shows you the pressure being generated by the bag. If the airway is blocked, the gauge will register, but no air will enter the lungs. You must observe chest movement as well.)

Decision

If . . .	Then . . .
You had the correct answers to at least 15 of the 17 questions . . .	Good. You are doing well. Go on to the next section.
You missed 3 or more . . .	Review the material carefully. The information is essential to your being able to ventilate an infant safely and effectively.

Ventilation Rate and Pressure

Up to this point, you have learned how to select and assemble a resuscitation bag and mask and how to check to be sure they are functioning properly. In addition, you have learned how to position the mask on the infant's face and how to test for an effective seal. Here you will learn how rapidly to squeeze the bag and what pressures should be used with various infants. In order for positive-pressure ventilation to be effective, it must be delivered at a proper rate and a proper pressure.

Ventilation Rate

Ventilation of the infant should be performed at a rate of *40–60 per minute.*

Practice

Practice squeezing the bag at a rate of 40–60. You can do this with or without a manikin. But you need a resuscitation bag and a clock with a second hand to time yourself.

Rate of 40–60 = 10–15 breaths in 15 seconds

If you had trouble maintaining a rate of 40–60, it may help for you to say to yourself as you ventilate an infant:

"squeeze,	two, (release)	three, (release)	squeeze"

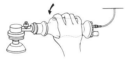 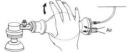 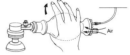 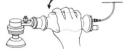

If you squeeze the bag on "squeeze," and release while you say "two, three," you will probably find you are ventilating at a proper rate.

Ventilation Pressure

The pressure needed to inflate the lungs will vary, depending on the infant's size, condition of the lungs, and whether the infant has previously taken a breath.

First breath	The initial lung inflation following delivery may require 30–40 cm H_2O pressure.
Succeeding breaths	Pressure of 15–20 is often adequate after the first breath.
Pulmonary disease*	Infants with respiratory conditions that decrease lung compliance may require 20–40 cm H_2O pressure.

*The result of respiratory diseases in which some of the alveoli are collapsed, making the lungs difficult to expand (e.g., hyaline membrane disease, meconium aspiration).

Practice

If your bag has a pressure gauge, you can practice ventilating at the recommended pressures:

- 15–20 (infant with normal lungs)
- 30–40 (the initial breath following delivery)
- 20–40 (infants with pulmonary disease)

If you have a pressure-release valve rather than a gauge, you cannot practice ventilating at specific pressures. You should use pressures that produce a slight rise and fall of the chest without activating the pressure-release valve.

Note:

Now that you have learned how to form a seal and ventilate at appropriate rates and pressures, let's take a look at two procedures that might be necessary, under some circumstances, to effectively and safely ventilate an infant. These are:

- Inserting an orogastric tube, and
- Using an oral airway.

Orogastric Catheter

Infants requiring positive-pressure ventilation with a bag and mask for longer than *2 minutes* should have an orogastric tube inserted and left in place *during ventilation.* Here you will learn the importance of an orogastric tube in preventing distention of the stomach and intestines and preventing aspiration of gastric contents.

Effect of Ventilation

During bag-and-mask ventilation, air is forced into the oropharynx, where it is free to enter both the trachea and the esophagus. Proper positioning of the infant will force most of the air into the trachea and the lungs. However, some air may enter the esophagus and be forced into the stomach.

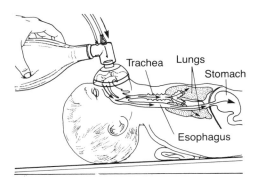

Distention

Air forced into the stomach interferes with ventilation in the following ways:
• Air in the stomach puts pressure on the diaphragm, preventing full expansion of the lungs.
• Air in the stomach may cause regurgitation of gastric contents, which can then be aspirated during bag-and-mask resuscitation.
• Air in the stomach travels into the bowel, producing abdominal distention for several hours. This puts pressure on the diaphragm and makes it more difficult for the infant to breathe.

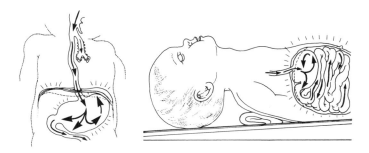

The problems related to gastric/abdominal distention and aspiration of gastric contents can be prevented by inserting an orogastric tube, suctioning gastric contents, and leaving the gastric tube in place to act as a vent for air throughout the remainder of the resuscitation.

Procedure

The equipment you will need in using an orogastric catheter during ventilation includes:

- 8 Fr. feeding tube
- 20-cc syringe

If you have not had experience in inserting an orogastric catheter and suctioning the stomach of a neonate, see your instructor or supervisor to arrange for supervised practice.

Major Points

The major steps in the procedure are:

1. Always measure the length of the catheter you want to insert. It must be long enough to reach the stomach, but not so long as to perforate it. The length of the inserted catheter should be equal to *the distance from the bridge of the nose to the earlobe and from the earlobe to the xiphoid process* (the lower tip of the sternum). To minimize interruption of ventilation, measurement of the orogastric tube can be approximated with the mask in place.

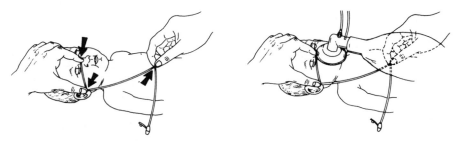

2. Insert the catheter *through the mouth* rather than the nose. The nose should be left open for ventilation. (Ventilation can be resumed as soon as the catheter has been placed.)

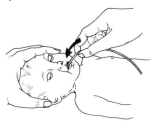

3. Once the catheter is inserted the desired distance, attach a 20-cc syringe and quickly, but gently, remove the gastric contents.

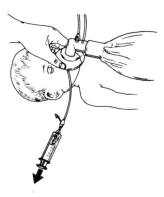

4. Remove the syringe from the catheter, and leave the end of the catheter *open* to provide a vent for air entering the stomach.

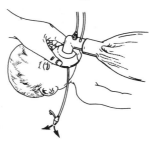

5. Tape the catheter to the infant's cheek to ensure that the tip remains in the stomach and is not pulled back into the esophagus.

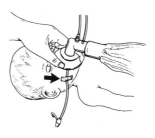

Note: The catheter will not interfere with the mask-to-face seal if an 8 Fr. feeding tube is used and the tube exits from the side of the mask over the soft area of the infant's cheek. A larger catheter may make it difficult to attain a seal. A smaller catheter can easily become occluded by secretions.

Oral Airway

Oral airways are *rarely* used for neonates during bag-and-mask ventilation. However, they must be readily available for use in the unusual circumstance when an infant has nasal obstruction or when the tongue blocks the airway.

Three conditions in which an oral airway may be required during ventilation are:

- Bilateral choanal atresia
- Pierre Robin syndrome
- When it is necessary to keep the mouth open to attain adequate ventilation

These situations are described below, along with the procedure for inserting an airway.

Choanal Atresia

Choanal atresia is a congenital blockage of one or both of the posterior nares by a membrane or bone.

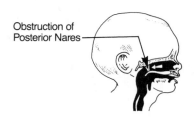

Obstruction of Posterior Nares

Infant with Choanal Atresia

If both nares are obstructed, an oral airway must be inserted immediately after birth and left in place until surgery is performed. Because young infants are nasal breathers, those with bilateral choanal atresia develop serious respiratory distress in the first few minutes of life.

The airway must remain in place whether ventilation is needed or not. It provides an unobstructed passage for air through the mouth.

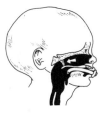

Unobstructed Oral Air Passage

Pierre Robin Syndrome

Pierre Robin syndrome is another abnormality that can require the use of an oral airway during ventilation. It is characterized by an abnormally small lower jaw. The tongue is of normal size, but, due to the small jaw, the tongue is easily forced against the posterior pharynx and can block the airway.

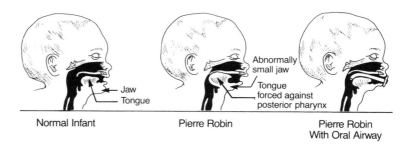

Normal Infant   Pierre Robin   Pierre Robin With Oral Airway

Ventilating With Mouth Open

Occasionally, when bag-and-mask ventilation does not lead to a rise of the chest, inserting an oral airway and ventilating through the mouth may produce the desired effect.

Procedure

Resuscitation trays should have at least two sizes of airways to accommodate premature and fullterm infants.

Selecting Airway

The airway should comfortably fit over the tongue, reaching the posterior pharynx with the flange just outside the lips. A device that is too small may force the tongue into the airway while one that is too large can cause injury.

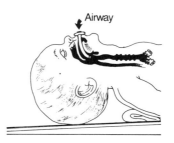

Inserting Airway

Insert the airway by opening the mouth and carefully directing the airway *over* the tongue. Be certain you are not forcing the tongue back as you insert the airway.

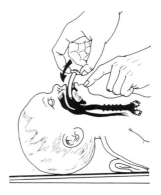

When inserting an airway in neonates, it is not necessary to initially reverse its position, as you might do in an older child or adult.

Practice Activity 3

Use this practice activity to test your knowledge of ventilation rates and pressures and the uses of an orogastric catheter and an oral airway.

Fill In

1. State the rate at which a neonate should be ventilated.
   _____–_____/minute

2. If an infant has not yet taken his or her first breath, you should ventilate with a pressure of _____–_____ cm H_2O.

3. If an infant's lungs are normal, what pressure should be used after the infant has taken his or her initial breath?
   _____–_____ cm H_2O

4. If an infant has pulmonary disease, what pressure range would be appropriate in ventilating the infant?
   _____–_____ cm H_2O

5–6. What are the two reasons for inserting an *orogastric tube* during bag-and-mask ventilation?

   • _____

   • _____

7. Name the three points used in measuring the length of a catheter for gastric suctioning.

   • _____

   • _____

   • _____

8. On the following diagram, draw lines to represent the position an *orogastric catheter* should be in at the time it is being measured.

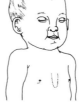

Multiple Choice

9. An *orogastric catheter* should be inserted if an infant requires ventilation with a bag and mask longer than what period of time?

   _____ **A.** 1 minute

   _____ **B.** 2 minutes

   _____ **C.** 3 minutes

   _____ **D.** 4 minutes

10–12. An *oral airway* may be required during bag-and-mask ventilation in which of the following situations? Place an "X" in front of each that applies.

_____ **A.** Infants with bilateral choanal atresia

_____ **B.** Whenever an infant is ventilated

_____ **C.** When ventilating an infant for longer than 2 minutes.

_____ **D.** When it is necessary to keep the mouth open to attain adequate ventilation

_____ **E.** Infants with a pneumothorax

_____ **F.** Infants with Pierre Robin syndrome

True/False

13. _____ Oral airways are rarely used in neonates during bag-and-mask ventilation.

14. _____ Airways for use with newborns come in one size, which is suitable for both premature and term infants.

15. _____ Choanal atresia refers to a congenital blockage of one or both of the posterior nares.

16. _____ An infant with Pierre Robin syndrome has an excessively large tongue.

17. _____ To relieve gastric distention in a neonate requiring prolonged ventilation, an 8 Fr. feeding tube should be inserted through the nose and into the stomach.

Practice Activity 3: Answers

Check your answers with those given here.

Fill In

1. 40—60

2. 30–40 cm H_2O

3. 15–20 cm H_2O

4. 20–40 cm H_2O

5–6. • To prevent gastric/abdominal distention
   • To suction gastric contents, thus preventing aspiration

7. • Bridge of the nose
   • Earlobe (must be the middle point listed)
   • Xiphoid process (tip of sternum)

8.

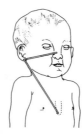

Multiple Choice

9. B

10–12. A, D, F

True/False

13. True

14. False — They come in several sizes. At least two sizes should be available to accommodate both premature and fullterm infants.

15. True

16. False — In Pierre Robin syndrome the tongue is of normal size, it is the jaw that is small. Airway obstruction can occur when the excessively small jaw forces the tongue back against the posterior pharynx.

17. False — The feeding tube should be inserted through the *mouth,* not through the nose.

Decision

If . . .	Then . . .
You had at least 15 correct . . .	Good work. Go on to the next section.
You missed more than 2 . . .	Review the text material, then try again to answer the questions you missed.

Posttest
Lesson 3B—
Use of a Resuscitation Bag and Mask: Ventilation

Name _____ Date _____

This posttest is designed to let you test yourself on your understanding of ventilating an infant. Follow the directions for each part.

Multiple Choice

1. Resuscitation bags for neonates should not exceed:

   _____ **A.** 240 mL

   _____ **B.** 500 mL

   _____ **C.** 750 mL

   _____ **D.** 1 liter (1000 mL)

Fill In

2. What concentration of oxygen should be used when ventilating an infant at birth?

   _____ to _____%

True/False

3. _____ When skilled in using a bag and mask, you should be able to ventilate an infant, using minimal pressure to hold the mask to the face.

4. _____ During ventilation, the mask should cover the mouth, nose, and tip of the chin, but not the eyes.

5. _____ Chest expansion indicates that you have an adequate mask/face seal.

Completion

6–8. You have suctioned, positioned, and given tactile stimulation to an infant who remains apneic. Using a bag and mask, you ventilate the infant two to three times, but you notice that the chest does not rise. What three basic problems should you consider as being possibly responsible for the lack of chest movement?

   • _____

   • _____

   • _____

   If you do not observe chest expansion, you should quickly remedy the situation so you can ventilate the baby. List, in order, the five steps you would go through to correct the problem.

   9. • _____

   10. • _____

   11. • _____

   12. • _____

   13. • _____

Multiple Choice

14. Which of the following are true of an infant being properly ventilated? Place an "X" in front of each that applies.

_____ **A.** You will see good chest expansion—the infant will appear to be taking a deep breath.

_____ **B.** The pressure gauge will register the appropriate ventilation pressure for the infant, although you may not see a rise and fall of the chest.

_____ **C.** You will see chest movement—the infant will appear to be taking a shallow or "easy" breath.

Fill In

15. State the rate at which a neonate should be ventilated.

_____–_____/minute

16. If an infant has not yet taken his or her first breath, you should ventilate with a pressure of _____–_____ cm H_2O.

17. If an infant's lungs are normal, what pressures should be used after the infant has taken his or her initial breath?
_____–_____ cm H_2O

18. If an infant has pulmonary disease, what pressure range would be appropriate in ventilating the infant?
_____–_____ cm H_2O

19–20. What are the two reasons for inserting an *orogastric tube* during bag-and-mask ventilation?

• _____

• _____

Multiple Choice

21. An *orogastric catheter* should be inserted if an infant requires ventilation with a bag and mask longer than what period of time?

_____ **A.** 1 minute

_____ **B.** 2 minutes

_____ **C.** 3 minutes

_____ **D.** 4 minutes

22–24. An *oral airway* may be indicated during bag-and-mask ventilation in which of the following situations? Place an "X" in front of each that applies.

_____ **A.** When an infant has bilateral choanal atresia

_____ **B.** Whenever an infant is ventilated

_____ **C.** When ventilating an infant for longer than 2 minutes

_____ **D.** When it is necessary to keep the mouth open to attain adequate ventilation

_____ **E.** When an infant has a pneumothorax

_____ **F.** When an infant has Pierre Robin syndrome

Lesson 3B Posttest: Answers

Check your answers with those given here.

Multiple Choice

1. C

Fill In

2. 90–100%

True/False

3. True

4. True

5. True

Completion

6–8. • Inadequate seal
   • Blocked airway
   • Not enough pressure

9. • Reapply mask to face
10. • Reposition the head
11. • Check for secretions, suction if necessary
12. • Ventilate with infant's mouth slightly open
13. • Increase pressure

Multiple Choice

14. <u>X</u> **C.** You will see chest movement—the infant will appear to be taking a shallow or "easy" breath.
   (If you answered **B**, remember that the pressure gauge shows you the pressure being generated by the bag. If the airway is blocked, the gauge will register, but no air will enter the lungs. You must observe chest movement as well.)

Fill In

15. 40

16. 30–40 cm H_2O

17. 15–20 cm H_2O

18. 20–40 cm H_2O

19–20. • To prevent gastric/abdominal distention
   • To suction gastric contents, thus preventing aspiration

Multiple Choice

21. B

22–24. A, D, F

Decision

If . . .	Then . . .
You answered 22 or more of the questions correctly . . .	You have done well. Go on to the performance checklist, and practice the indicated skills.
You missed 3 or more . . .	Go back and review the text material before going on to the performance checklist.

Performance Checklist
Lesson 3B—
Use of a Resuscitation Bag and Mask: Ventilation

Instructor: The participant should be instructed to talk through the procedure as it is demonstrated. Judge the performance of each step carried out, and check (✔) the box when the action is completed correctly. If done incorrectly, circle the box so that you can discuss that step later.

An infant resuscitation manikin must be used for the demonstration. You will need to provide information, at several points, concerning the condition of the "infant." This allows you to check the participant's ability to make correct decisions and take appropriate action based on those decisions.

To successfully complete this checklist, the participant should be able to **perform all the steps and make all the correct decisions in the procedure.**

Equipment and Supplies

Infant resuscitation manikin
Resuscitation bag and masks (several sizes)
Pressure gauge, if used
Oxygen reservoir, if using a self-inflating bag
Oxygen equipment:
    Oxygen source
    Flowmeter
    Tubing
    Blender, if used
Infant oral airways
8 Fr. feeding tube and 20-cc syringe
Adhesive tape—1/2" x 2"
Clock with second hand
Bulb syringe
Shoulder roll

Performance Checklist
Lesson 3B —
Use of a Resuscitation Bag and Mask: Ventilation

Name _____ Instructor _____ Date _____

Equipment Situation:

"Prepare and test the equipment you would need to provide PPV with a bag and mask to an infant of approximately _____ grams."

☐ **1. Selects bag and connects to oxygen source**
  • Capable of delivering 90–100% O_2?

☐ **2. Selects mask**
  • Correct size?

☐ **3. Tests bag**
  • Good pressure?
  • Pressure-release valve working?
  • Valve assembly present and functioning?
  • Pressure gauge (if any) working?
  (If bag is not working properly, obtains and tests another)

Patient Situation:

"An infant has just been born, provided thermal management, positioned, suctioned, and given tactile stimulation. The infant is apneic. Establish ventilation in this infant using a bag and mask."

☐ **4. Checks infant's position**
  • Head extended slightly?
  • Slight Trendelenburg?

☐ **5. Positions bag and mask properly on infant**

☐ **6. Checks seal** (Gives two or three ventilations at appropriate pressure and observes for chest movement)

☐ **Rise**

☐ **No Rise**

☐ Checks for inadequate seal
  • Reapplies face mask

Yes ◇ Rise?

No

Easy breath

☐ Checks for blocked airway
  • Repositions head
  • Checks for secretions
  • Ventilates with mouth slightly open

Yes ◇ Rise?

No

☐ Increases ventilation pressure

○

☐ **7. Ventilates for 15-30 seconds**
  • Rate: 40–60 times/minute
  • Pressure: A slight rise and fall of chest attained

Instructor: "Demonstrate how you would insert and manage an orogastric catheter in an infant requiring ventilation."

☐ **8. Uses correct procedure**
- Measures catheter correctly
- Inserts catheter through mouth the proper distance
- Suctions gastric contents
- Leaves catheter end open
- Tapes catheter to cheek

Overall

☐ Speed—no undue delays

☐ Handling of infant was safe, without trauma

☐ Ventilated with appropriate pressure

☐ Avoided using excessive pressure on mask

Use of a Resuscitation Bag and Mask: Ventilation as Part of the Resuscitation Procedure

Contents

Use of a Resuscitation Bag and Mask: Ventilation as Part of the Resuscitation Procedure

Overview of Lesson 3C

The single most important procedure used in resuscitating neonates is positive-pressure ventilation. In the majority of cases, proper oxygenation can be restored with the bag and mask *if* it is used promptly by a skilled operator familiar with the equipment and its application.

When ventilation is delayed by prolonged use of tactile stimulation or attempts at intubation, the infant becomes increasingly more asphyxiated. The arterial oxygen tension (PaO_2), heart rate, and blood pressure fall, and additional resuscitative measures such as chest compressions and medications may be required to stabilize the infant.

Not only is it essential to become skilled in using a bag and mask, but it is also important to know how the use of a bag and mask fits in with the other procedures that might be indicated in the management of the asphyxiated newborn.

In this lesson, you will learn when to begin positive-pressure ventilation, when it can be safely discontinued, and when, in addition to ventilation, chest compressions should be used.

Performance Checklist

The performance checklist will be used by your instructor or supervisor to make sure that you are able to perform all the steps of the bag-and-mask ventilation procedure correctly and in the proper order. This checklist will also serve as a guide to help you in practicing the procedure.

Prerequisites

Before you study this lesson, be sure you have completed the previous two parts of this lesson—Parts A and B. To begin this lesson, you must already:

- Know how to prepare the equipment you will use with bag-and-mask ventilation.
- Be able to easily ventilate the manikin, using a correct rate and pressure.
- Feel comfortable in using an orogastric catheter as a vent for air and to suction gastric contents.

If you need additional practice or assistance, see your instructor.

Equipment Needed

The following is a summary list of the equipment you will need.

Bag

Resuscitation bag
- Pressure gauge, if one is used
- Oxygen reservoir, if a self-inflating bag is used

Masks

Face masks (appropriate size for use with manikin)

Oxygen Equipment

Oxygen source (oxygen tank or a wall oxygen outlet)
Flowmeter
Oxygen tubing
Air/oxygen blender, if used in your area

Orogastric Catheter and Syringe

8 Fr. feeding tube and 20-cc syringe

Tape

Adhesive tape — 1/2" x 2"

Manikin

For this part of the lesson a manikin will be required.

Objectives

Knowledge

After completing Part C, you will be expected to:

- State two indications for providing positive-pressure ventilation.
- State how long you should initially ventilate an infant before checking the heart rate.
- Identify when chest compressions should be initiated in an infant receiving positive-pressure ventilation.
- When given a 6-second heart rate, indicate whether the 1-minute heart rate is: below 60, between 60 and 100, or greater than 100.
- List three signs that indicate that a neonate's condition is improving.
- When given case situations, identify whether tactile stimulation, positive-pressure ventilation, or chest compression is indicated.
- State the equipment that should be used to provide positive-pressure ventilation to an infant suspected of having a diaphragmatic hernia.

Clinical

Your performance will be measured using the performance checklist at the end of this lesson. You will be expected to:

- Perform bag-and-mask ventilation on an infant resuscitation manikin, using the described technique.
- When given clinical data, make the correct decisions in the resuscitation procedure.

Decision Table

If . . .	Then . . .
You feel you can pass a test on the objectives . . .	Turn to the posttest.
You wish to know more before trying the posttest . . .	Go on to the next page and begin the lesson.

Indications

Positive-pressure ventilation should be initiated as soon as it is indicated. To delay ventilating an infant in whom it is indicated will only prolong the resuscitative efforts and place the infant at risk for further damage.

Preceding Events

Immediately after birth the infant should be:
• Placed under a radiant warmer,
• Wiped dry,
• Properly positioned,
• Suctioned, and
• Provided with tactile stimulation.

Most often, it is only after the infant has reached this point that a decision regarding positive-pressure ventilation can be made.

Two Indications for Ventilation

After tactile stimulation, positive-pressure ventilation should be initiated in any infant who is apneic or gasping or whose respirations are at any time insufficient to maintain a heart rate above 100 beats/minute. Thus, positive-pressure ventilation should begin when:
• Infant is apneic or gasping,
   or
• Heart rate is less than 100 beats/min.

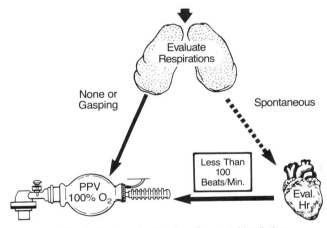

Two Indications for Positive-Pressure Ventilation

Bag and Mask Versus Bag and Endotracheal Tube

Positive-pressure ventilation can be provided with either a bag and mask or a bag and endotracheal tube. Although some infants cannot be adequately ventilated with a bag and mask, in most, proper use of a bag and mask can provide positive-pressure ventilation in an effective and timely manner. While some experienced individuals prefer to insert an endotracheal tube when PPV is required, valuable time can be wasted and trauma can be induced by an unskilled intubation, expecially if several attempts are made.

Exception to Using a Mask

If an infant is suspected of having a diaphragmatic hernia, PPV should be provided via an endotracheal tube. In a diaphragmatic hernia, abdominal organs (i.e., stomach, bowel) are displaced into the chest, compressing the heart and lungs. Ventilating with an endotracheal tube rather than a mask prevents air from entering and distending the gastrointestinal tract, thus further compromising ventilation.

PPV via mask   PPV via ET Tube

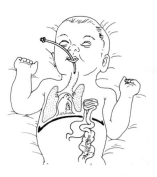

Outline of the Procedure

This final part of the lesson teaches you when to use a bag and mask and how to monitor the infant to evaluate the effectiveness of the ventilation. Also included is information on the decisions to be made on the basis of the infant's heart rate. The procedure and the sequence of the steps involved follow:
- Select and check the equipment.
- Obtain an effective seal.
- Ventilate the infant.
- Monitor the heart rate.
- Make correct decisions based on the infant's heart rate.

Select Equipment

The first step in the ventilation procedure is selecting the appropriate equipment.
- Obtain a resuscitation bag and connect it to an oxygen source.
- Select a mask of the correct size and attach it to the bag.
- Select an airway if one is indicated.

Check Bag

Next, quickly test your bag to see if it functions properly. If it does not function as it should, get another bag and test it.

Check Infant's Position

Now check the infant's position. The neck should be slightly extended.

Position Mask, Check Seal

Form a seal between the mask and the infant's face.
Check the seal by ventilating two or three times and observing for a rise of the chest.

Ventilate Infant 15-30 Seconds

Once a seal is ensured and chest movement is present, give an initial 15- to 30-second period of ventilation. As you ventilate, keep the proper rate and pressures in mind:

Rate

Rate
- 40–60 per minute

Pressures

Although you will ventilate with the lowest pressure required to move the chest, initial breaths may require pressures as high as 40 cm of water. Subsequent breaths usually require less pressure.

Pressures
- Initial breath after delivery   30–40 cm H_2O
- Normal lungs   15–20 cm H_2O
- Diseased lungs   20–40 cm H_2O

**Evaluate
Heart Rate**

After the infant has been ventilated for 15–30 seconds, check the heart rate. What you do next is based on the heart rate.

Decisions

HR Above 100

1. If the heart rate is above 100 beats/minute and the infant has spontaneous respirations, discontinue positive-pressure ventilation. However, if there are no spontaneous respirations, ventilation must be continued.

*HR 60–100
and Increasing*

2. If the heart rate is 60–100 and *increasing:*
   • Continue ventilation.

*HR 60–100 and
Not Increasing*

3. If the heart rate is 60–100 and *not increasing:*
   • Continue ventilation—checking adequacy of ventilation.
      • Is chest moving properly/Are breath sounds adequate?
      • Is 100% oxygen being administered?
   • If heart rate is less than 80 beats/minute, start chest compressions.

HR Below 60

4. If the heart rate is below 60 beats per minute:
   • Continue ventilation—checking adequacy of ventilation.
      • Is chest moving properly/Are breath sounds adequate?
      • Is 100% oxygen being administered?
   • Immediately begin chest compressions.

Stop Points

If continued ventilation is indicated, continue to monitor the heart rate and respirations until:

The heart rate and respirations reach acceptable levels.

If heart rate and respirations do not reach acceptable levels with bag and mask ventilation, it will be necessary to provide additional resuscitative assistance, i.e., chest compressions, endotracheal intubation, and administration of medications.

Evaluating Heart Rate

After ventilating the infant for the initial 15–30 seconds, you must check the infant's heart rate. Here you will learn how this can be done quickly.

Detecting Heartbeat

The infant's heart rate can be detected in either of two ways:
- Listening to the apical beat with a stethoscope;
- Feeling the umbilical or brachial pulse.

If there is a second person available or the baby is on a cardiac monitor, the heart rate can be checked while you are ventilating. If you do not have a second person or monitor to assist you, then you must stop ventilating the infant to check the heart rate.

Determining Heart Rate

To minimize the time lost, the heart rate can be determined in just 6 seconds. If you listen to the heartbeat for 6 seconds and multiply the number by 10, you will have an approximation of the 1-minute heart rate. For example, if the heart beats 8 times in 6 seconds, the 1-minute heart rate is approximately 80.

At first it may seem strange to count the heart rate for such a short period of time. Once you learn to do so, you will find it will save valuable time, allowing you to make decisions quickly when managing an infant requiring resuscitation.

At this point in the resuscitative effort, you only need to know if the heart rate is:
- Below 60
- Between 60 and 100, or
- Above 100

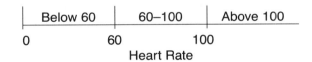

In the next section, you will learn the interventions appropriate for infants in each of these three heart-rate categories.

Practice

It is likely that you are not used to counting the heartbeat for just 6 seconds. You should therefore practice doing so on healthy infants or yourself, so that when managing an asphyxiated infant, counting for 6 seconds and multiplying by 10 is automatic.

Practice Activity 1

Use this practice activity to test your knowledge of the material presented thus far in this lesson.

Fill In

1—2. List the two indications for positive-pressure ventilation.

* _____

* _____

3. What equipment should be used in providing PPV to an infant suspected of having a diaphragmatic hernia?

_____

Matching

For each of the 6-second heart rates given below, indicate whether the 1-minute heart rate is below 60, between 60 and 100, or above 100.

6-second H.R.

4. 11 _____

5. 6 _____

6. 8 _____

7. 4 _____

8. 14 _____

9. 7 _____

1-minute H.R.

A. Below 60

B. Between 60 and 100

C. Above 100

Practice Activity 1: Answers

Check your answers with those given here.

Fill In

1–2. • Apnea/gasping respirations
• Heart rate of less than 100

3. Endotracheal tube (and bag)

Matching

4. C

5. B

6. B

7. A

8. C

9. B

Decision

If . . .	Then . . .
You answered all of the questions correctly . . .	Go on to the next section.
You missed any questions . . .	Review the material that gave you trouble.

Heart Rate Decisions

The decisions you make regarding care are based on the three categories of heart rate just studied. Let's look at each decision.

Above 100

If the infant has a heart rate above 100 beats/minute, he or she is nearing a normal heart rate. If the infant begins breathing spontaneously, PPV can be interrupted to assess adequacy of ventilation. After discontinuing PPV, an initial period of free-flow oxygen should always be provided. The oxygen may be withdrawn slowly if the infant remains pink.

Gentle tactile stimulation may be helpful in supporting early respiratory efforts. The rate and depth of infants' respirations frequently increase in response to cutaneous stimulation.

Thus, if after a period of positive-pressure ventilation an infant begins to breathe spontaneously, you should:

- Discontinue PPV
- Provide an initial period of free-flow oxygen
- Provide gentle tactile stimulation as necessary

If, however, adequate spontaneous respirations are not maintained:

- Continue PPV

Between 60 and 100

60–100 and _Increasing_

60–100 and _Not Increasing_

If an infant's heart rate is between 60 and 100 beats/minute, try to determine if the heart rate is increasing. To determine if the heart rate is increasing (or falling), you may have to listen for more than 6 seconds.

If the heart rate is starting to increase:

- Continue ventilation.

If the infant's heart rate is in the range of 60–100, but is _not increasing:_

- Continue ventilation—checking adequacy of ventilation.
    - Is chest movement sufficient/Are breath sounds adequate?
    - Is 100% oxygen being administered?
- _If HR is less than 80,_ initiate chest compressions. (A second person must be present to initiate chest compressions.)

Below 60

A neonate with a 6-second heart rate below 6 (60/minute) after an initial period of ventilation with 100% oxygen is in serious trouble. In that case:

- Continue ventilation—checking adequacy of ventilation.
    - Is chest movement sufficient/Are breath sounds adequate?
    - Is 100% oxygen being administered?
- _Immediately_ begin chest compressions.

Flow Diagram

The following diagram summarizes the heart-rate decisions.

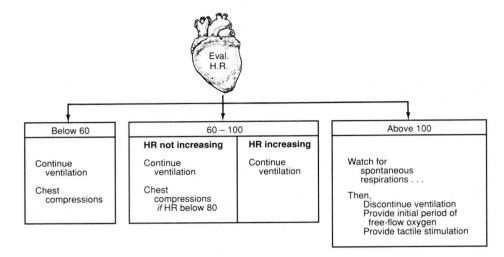

Below 60	60 – 100		Above 100
	HR not increasing	**HR increasing**	
Continue ventilation	Continue ventilation	Continue ventilation	Watch for spontaneous respirations . . .
Chest compressions	Chest compressions *if* HR below 80		Then, Discontinue ventilation Provide initial period of free-flow oxygen Provide tactile stimulation

Improvement

Improvement in the neonate is indicated by three signs:
• Increasing heart rate,
• Spontaneous respirations, and
• Improving color.

The steps you go through will depend upon the degree of improvement in the infant's condition.

Signs of Improvement

Heart Rate

As the heart rate keeps increasing toward normal, you should continue ventilating the baby at a rate of 40–60 breaths per minute. Monitor the rise of the chest to prevent overinflation or underinflation of the lungs.

When the heart rate stabilizes above 100 beats per minute, stop ventilating, but continue to provide a high-oxygen environment and observe whether the baby can sustain adequate spontaneous respirations.

Respirations

If the infant is breathing spontaneously and the heart rate has reached an acceptable level, you may provide gentle tactile stimulation until the rate and depth of respirations are normal. Continue to monitor the infant to determine whether or not adequate respirations are maintained.

Color

With improvement, the infant should become pink.

Deterioration

We have analyzed the steps to be taken if a neonate's condition improves. Now let's consider the infant who *does not* improve.

Initial Actions

If, with continued assisted ventilation, the infant's condition continues to deteriorate or fails to improve, check adequacy of ventilation and start chest compressions if the heart rate is less than 80 beats/minute.

Check Adequacy of Ventilation

Is chest movement adequate?

Check for adequacy of chest expansion and use a stethoscope to listen for bilateral breath sounds.

- Is the face/mask seal tight?
- Is the airway blocked due to improper head position or secretions in the nose, mouth, or pharynx?
- Is adequate pressure being used?
- Is air in the stomach interfering with chest expansion?

Is 100% oxygen being administered?

- Is the oxygen tubing attached to the bag *and* to the flowmeter?
- If using a blender, is it set at 100%?
- If using a self-inflating bag, is the oxygen reservoir attached?
- If using a tank (rather than wall oxygen), is there oxygen in the tank?

These all seem obvious. However, in the urgency created by an infant needing resuscitation, some of these points may be overlooked.

An individual skilled in resuscitation but not actively involved can play a vital role by observing problems and taking remedial action.

Chest Compressions

Provide chest compressions if indicated.

If, despite assisted ventilation, the heart rate remains below 80 beats/minute, chest compressions should be initiated.

Additional Procedures

If the infant's condition continues to deteriorate or fails to improve despite assisted ventilation and chest compressions, the infant may require:

- Endotracheal intubation
- Medications

Consider Intubation

A bag and mask is usually effective for neonatal ventilation. However, if ventilation with bag and mask is ineffective, the infant should be intubated. In addition, when the need for prolonged ventilation is anticipated, it is often easier to continue the ventilation if the infant is intubated.

Thus, there are two main reasons for switching to ventilation via an endotracheal tube:

- **For effectiveness** — If you have any reason to believe that bag-and-mask ventilation is not providing effective ventilation;
- **For convenience** — If ventilation is to be continued for a prolonged period of time.

Administer Medications

A discussion of medications, their indication and dosage, is presented in Lesson 6.

Recap

If an infant's condition continues to deteriorate or if, despite continued ventilation, it fails to improve (as evidenced by a falling heart rate or a heart rate that fails to increase), these steps should be taken:

- Continue ventilation, and
- Start chest compressions if the heart rate is less than 80 beats/min.
- Call for additional help if needed.

If positive-pressure ventilation and chest compressions do not lead to improvement:

- Consider intubation.
- Consider medications.

Practice Activity 2

Use this practice activity to test your knowledge of some key concepts, including heart-rate decisions.

Fill In

1–3. What three signs indicate that a neonate who has required resuscitation is improving?

- _____

- _____

- _____

4. After obtaining a good face/mask seal, approximately how long should you initially ventilate an infant before checking the heart rate?

_____

5–11. Each of the heart rates below was obtained after an *initial* period of positive-pressure ventilation. Place a (✔) in the appropriate column(s) to identify interventions that should be initiated for each case.

1-minute Heart Rate	Tactile Stim.	Continue PPV	D/C PPV	Chest Compressions
30				
120 and spont. resp.				
70 and not increasing				
70 and increasing				
140 and no spont. resp.				

Practice Activity 2: Answers

Check your answers with those given here.

Fill In

1–3. • Increasing heart rate
• Spontaneous respirations
• Improving color

4. 15–30 seconds

5–11.

1-minute Heart Rate	Tactile Stim.	Continue PPV	D/C PPV	Chest Compressions
30		✔		✔
120 and spont. resp.	✔ optional		✔	
70 and not increasing		✔		✔
70 and increasing		✔		
140 and no spont. resp.	✔ optional	✔		

Note: Optional ✔'s are not scored.

Decision

If . . .	Then . . .
You missed 2 or fewer . . .	You did well. Go on to the next section.
You missed 3 or more . . .	Review the appropriate material, and try again to answer those questions.

Summary

This brief summary of bag-and-mask (positive-pressure) ventilation will serve as a reminder of the key points in the procedure. Before you go on to the posttest, however, you may want to review more thoroughly by going back to specific portions of this lesson.

Preparations

The need for possible resuscitation of a neonate should be anticipated.

Equipment

This means that all the necessary resuscitation equipment should be in working order and immediately available in the delivery room at all times. This equipment includes a resuscitation bag capable of providing 90–100% oxygen (anesthesia bag or self-inflating bag with oxygen reservoir) and neonatal masks of various sizes. An oxygen source must be readily available, along with a flowmeter and/or an oxygen blender and oxygen tubing. Suction equipment should include, at a minimum, a bulb syringe, suction tubing, mechanical suction, and appropriate sized catheters. A syringe and orogastric catheter, oral airway, and intubation equipment should be kept close at hand.

Infant

By the time an infant reaches the point of needing bag-and-mask ventilation, he or she has been placed under a radiant heater, dried, positioned, suctioned, and provided with tactile stimulation.

Bag-and-Mask Indications

Bag-and-mask ventilation is indicated any time an infant is apneic or gasping, or respirations cannot maintain a heart rate above 100 beats/ minute.

Select Equipment

The first step is to select the appropriate equipment:
• Obtain resuscitation bag and connect it to an oxygen source.
• Select a mask of the proper size.
• Quickly check the bag to be sure it functions properly (if you did not do so previously).

Check Infant's Position

The infant's neck should be slightly extended to assure an open airway.

Position Mask and Obtain Seal

Place the mask in position and check the seal by ventilating two or three times. Observe for an appropriate rise of the chest.

No Rise

If chest does not rise:

Action	Condition Corrected
1. Reapply mask	Inadequate seal
2. Reposition infant's head	Blocked airway
3. Check for secretions, suction if present	Blocked airway
4. Ventilate with mouth slightly open	Blocked airway
5. Increase pressure slightly	Inadequate pressure

If chest *still* does not rise, get a new bag, check it, and try again.

Normal Rise

When a normal rise of the chest is observed, begin ventilating.

Check Heart Rate

After the infant has received 15–30 seconds of ventilation with 100% oxygen, check the heart rate for 6 seconds. Is the heart rate below 60, between 60 and 100, or above 100 beats/minute? If it is between 60 and 100, note if it is increasing or not.

Heart Rate	Action
Above 100/min.	• If spontaneous respirations are present, provide tactile stimulation and monitor heart rate, respirations, and color • If not breathing or if gasping, continue ventilation
60–100/min. and increasing	• Continue ventilation
60–100/min. and *not* increasing	• Continue ventilation—check adequacy of ventilation • Begin chest compressions if HR below 80
Below 60/min.	• Continue to ventilate • Begin chest compressions

Signs of Improvement

There are three signs that indicate improvement in the condition of an infant undergoing resuscitation:
- Increasing heart rate,
- Spontaneous respirations, and
- Improving color.

Steps for Improvement

If the infant's condition fails to improve, take these steps:
- Continue ventilation—carefully check adequacy of ventilation.
- Initiate chest compressions if heart rate is below 80.
- Call for additional help if needed.

If PPV and chest compressions do not lead to improvement:
- Consider intubation of the trachea and administration of medications.

Note:

If ventilation continues for more than 2 minutes, an orogastric tube should be inserted as an air vent to relieve abdominal distention.

Posttest
Lesson 3C—
Use of a Resuscitation Bag and Mask: Procedure

Name _____ Date _____

Use this posttest to test your understanding of ventilation as part of the resuscitation procedure. Follow the directions for each part.

Fill In

1–2. List the two indications for positive-pressure ventilation.

• _____

• _____

Matching

For each of the 6-second heart rates given below, indicate whether the 1-minute heart rate is below 60, between 60 and 100, or above 100.

6-second H.R.

3. 5 _____

4. 2 _____

5. 11 _____

6. 8 _____

7. 15 _____

1-minute H.R.

A. Below 60

B. Between 60 and 100

C. Above 100

Fill In

8–14. Each of the heart rates below was obtained after an initial period of positive-pressure ventilation. Place a (✔) in the appropriate column(s) to identify interventions that should be initiated for each case.

1-minute Heart Rate	Tactile Stim.	Continue PPV	D/C PPV	Chest Compressions
70 and increasing				
120 and spont. resp.				
40				
140 and no spont. resp.				
70 and not increasing				

15–17. What three signs indicate that a neonate who has required resuscitation is improving?

- _____

- _____

- _____

18. After obtaining a good face/mask seal, approximately how long should you initially ventilate an infant before checking the heart rate?

_____

19. What equipment should be used in providing PPV to an infant suspected of having a diaphragmatic hernia?

_____

Lesson 3C Posttest: Answers

Check your answers with those given here.

Fill In

1–2. • Apnea/gasping respirations
• Heart rate of less than 100

Matching

3. A

4. A

5. C

6. B

7. C

Fill In

8–14.

1-minute Heart Rate	Tactile Stim.	Continue PPV	D/C PPV	Chest Compressions
70 and increasing		✔		
120 and spont. resp.	✔ optional		✔	
40		✔		✔
140 and no spont. resp.	✔ optional	✔		
70 and not increasing		✔		✔

Optional ✔'s are not scored.

15–17. • Increasing heart rate
• Spontaneous respirations
• Improving color

18. 15–30 seconds

19. Endotracheal tube (and bag)

Decision

If . . .	Then . . .
You missed no more than 2 . . .	You did well. Go on to the performance checklist.
You missed 3 or more . . .	Review the appropriate material before going on to the performance checklist.

Performance Checklist
Lesson 3C —
Use of a Resuscitation Bag and Mask: Procedure

Instructions

Instructor: The participant should be instructed to talk through the procedure as it is demonstrated. Judge the performance of each step carried out, and check (✓) the box when the action is completed correctly. If done incorrectly, circle the box so that you can discuss that step later.

An infant resuscitation manikin must be used for the demonstration. You will need to provide, at several points, information concerning the condition of the "infant." This allows you to check the participant's ability to make correct decisions and take appropriate action based on those decisions.

To successfully complete this checklist, the participant should be able to **perform all the steps and make all the correct decisions in the procedure.**

Equipment and Supplies

Infant resuscitation manikin
Resuscitation bag and masks (several sizes)
Pressure gauge, if used
Oxygen reservoir, if using a self-inflating bag
Oxygen equipment
    Oxygen source
    Flowmeter
    Tubing
    Blender, if used
Stethoscope
8 Fr. feeding tube and 20-cc syringe
Adhesive tape — 1/2" x 2"
Clock with second hand
Bulb syringe
Shoulder roll

Performance Checklist
Lesson 3C—
Use of a Resuscitation Bag and Mask: Procedure

Name _____ Instructor _____ Date _____

Equipment Situation:

"Prepare and test the equipment you need to provide PPV with a bag and mask to an infant of approximately _____ grams."

☐ **1. Selects bag and connects to oxygen source**
• Capable of delivering 90–100% O_2?

☐ **2. Selects mask**
• Correct size?

☐ **3. Tests bag**
• Good pressure?
• Pressure-release valve working?
• Valve assembly present and functioning?
• Pressure gauge (if any) working?
(If bag is not working properly, obtains and tests another)

Patient Situation:

"An infant has just been born, provided thermal management, positioned, suctioned, and given tactile stimulation. The infant is apneic. Establish ventilation in this infant using a bag and mask."

☐ **4. Checks infant's position**
• Head extended slightly?
• Slight Trendelenburg?

☐ **5. Positions bag and mask properly on infant**

☐ **6. Checks seal** (Gives two or three ventilations at appropriate pressure and observes for chest movement)

☐ **Rise**

☐ **No Rise**

☐ Checks for inadequate seal
• Reapplies face mask

◇ Rise? — Yes / No

Easy breath

☐ Checks for blocked airway
• Repositions head
• Checks for secretions
• Ventilates with mouth slightly open

◇ Rise? — Yes / No

☐ Increases ventilation pressure

○

☐ **7. Ventilates for 15-30 seconds**
• Rate: 40–60 times/minute
• Pressure: A slight rise and fall of chest attained

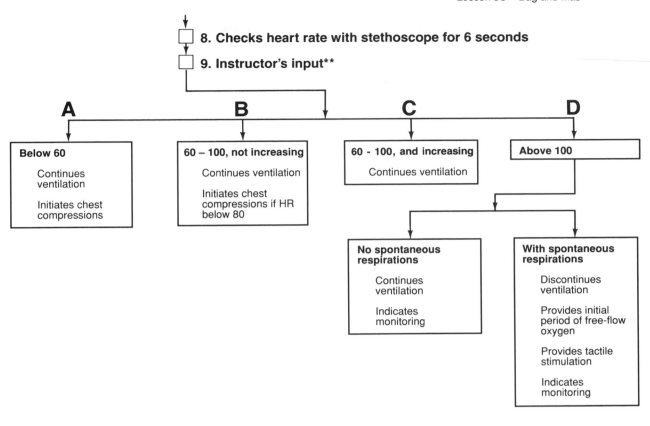

□ **8. Checks heart rate with stethoscope for 6 seconds**

□ **9. Instructor's input****

A | **B** | **C** | **D**

Below 60

Continues ventilation

Initiates chest compressions

60 – 100, not increasing

Continues ventilation

Initiates chest compressions if HR below 80

60 - 100, and increasing

Continues ventilation

Above 100

No spontaneous respirations

Continues ventilation

Indicates monitoring

With spontaneous respirations

Discontinues ventilation

Provides initial period of free-flow oxygen

Provides tactile stimulation

Indicates monitoring

**Present the five situations (A, B, C, and both parts of D) separately, and evaluate the trainee's response for each one.

Overall

□ Speed — no undue delays

□ Handling of infant was safe, with no trauma produced

□ Ventilated at appropriate rate (40–60/min)

□ Ventilated with appropriate pressure

□ Avoided using excessive pressure on mask

□ If ventilation continued longer than 2 minutes, an orogastric tube was inserted

Chest Compressions Lesson 4

Contents

Chest Compressions   Lesson 4

Introduction to Lesson 4

When a newborn infant is asphyxiated, serious effects on the infant's heart can occur as a result of the hypoxemia. In such cases, both the heart rate and myocardial contractility are reduced, resulting in bradycardia and less powerful contractions. The effect is a diminished flow of blood and therefore a diminished oxygen supply to vital tissues.

Chest compressions provide an artificial heart beat, thus restoring the circulation at a diminished, but life-sustaining, level. Positive-pressure ventilation must always accompany chest compressions so that the circulating blood will be oxygenated.

Overview of Lesson

This lesson is the fourth in the *Neonatal Resuscitation* series. The first three lessons were: "An Introduction to the Program," "Initial Steps in Resuscitation," and "Use of a Resuscitation Bag and Mask." Those lessons presented background information important to anyone responsible for chest compressions.

Because an infant in need of chest compressions will also be receiving positive-pressure ventilation, the procedure taught here is a two-person procedure: one person ventilates, and the other performs chest compressions.

In this lesson you will learn how to perform chest compressions on an infant who is receiving positive-pressure ventilation. You will also learn to ventilate an infant, using a bag and mask, while chest compressions are being performed.

After giving you an overview of chest compressions and the indications for initiating them, this lesson will teach the necessary information and skills related to positioning of the infant, chest compressions, and evaluation of the infant's heart rate. A review of the procedure, a case study, and a summary will assist you in remembering and applying the concepts and principles presented in the lesson. A performance checklist is provided for your use in practicing the procedure. The instructor will also use the checklist to verify that you are adequately able to perform all steps in the procedure.

Prerequisites

This lesson builds on the knowledge and skills you have acquired from other lessons in this series. Before you begin this lesson, you should be certain that you have mastered the knowledge and skills needed to effectively use a resuscitation bag and mask.

Objectives

Knowledge

When you finish this lesson, you will be asked to:

- Describe the situation and two heart-rate indications for initiating chest compressions on a neonate.
- Locate on a diagram of an infant's chest the area to be compressed during chest compressions.
- State the procedure that should always accompany chest compressions.
- For each of the two techniques taught, state the parts of the hand that should be used when compressing the infant's chest.

- State the rate at which chest compressions should be performed on a neonate.
- State the *rate* at which ventilation should be provided to a newborn undergoing chest compressions.
- When given a case study involving chest compressions, state the appropriate steps to be taken.
- State when chest compressions should be discontinued.
- List two complications that can result from chest compressions.

Performance

After instruction and practice on an infant resuscitation manikin, you must be able to do both the compression portion and the ventilation portion of this procedure. Specifically, you should be able to:

- Perform chest compressions as specified in this lesson (using both techniques) at a rate of 120/minute on an infant-size resuscitation manikin while the manikin is being ventilated with a bag and mask.
- Perform bag-and-mask ventilation at a rate of 40–60/minute while another person is performing chest compressions on the manikin at a rate of 120/ minute.

Decision Table

If . . .	Then . . .
You feel you can pass a test on these objectives . . .	Turn to the posttest on page 4-34.
You wish to know more before attempting the test . . .	Continue on the next page.

Overview of Chest Compressions

In the introductory lesson to this *Neonatal Resuscitation* program, we reviewed the ABCs — the basic principles — of cardiopulmonary resuscitation:

A — Open the *airway*.

B — Initiate *breathing*.

C — Assure *circulation*.

Chest compressions provide circulation, the "C" of these ABCs. The purpose of chest compression is to assure that the infant maintains a minimal, life-sustaining *circulation*.

Why Perform Chest Compressions?

The heart circulates blood throughout the body, delivering oxygen to vital organs. When an infant has suffered hypoxia, the heart not only slows in rate, but myocardial contractility is decreased. As a result, there is a diminished flow of blood and oxygen to the vital organs. The decreased supply of oxygen to these tissues can lead to irreparable damage to the brain, heart, kidneys, and bowel. Chest compressions are used to temporarily increase circulation and oxygen delivery.

Chest compressions must always be accompanied by ventilation with 100% oxygen. Ventilation must be performed to assure that the blood being circulated during chest compressions is oxygenated.

What is Chest Compression?

Chest compression, sometimes referred to as *external cardiac massage*, consists of rhythmic compressions of the sternum that:

• Compress the heart against the spine,

• Increase the intrathoracic pressure, and

• Circulate blood to the vital organs of the body.

The heart lies in the chest, between the sternum and the spine. Compressing the sternum compresses the heart and increases the pressure in the chest, causing blood to be pumped into the arteries. When pressure on the sternum is released, blood enters the heart from the veins.

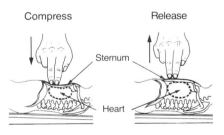

Compress | Release | Sternum | Heart

Practicing Chest Compressions

Successful performance of chest compressions requires a considerable amount of practice. One of the best ways to get this practice is to use an infant-size manikin. If you have such a manikin available, you may wish to use it for practicing chest compressions as you read this lesson. **Under no circumstances should you attempt to practice on a live infant.**

Indications for Chest Compressions

An adequate heart rate is necessary for effective cardiac output. Most of the time, ventilation alone with 100% oxygen will be sufficient to raise the infant's heart rate to an adequate level. If, despite being ventilated with 100% oxygen, an infant fails to achieve an adequate heart rate, chest compressions must be performed.

Initial Period of PPV

In a newborn, bradycardia usually results from a lack of proper oxygenation. In most infants with bradycardia, the heart rate begins to improve as soon as adequate ventilation with 100% oxygen is established.

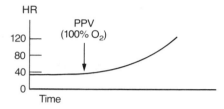

Therefore, the decision to begin chest compressions should be based on the heart rate obtained after 15–30 seconds of positive-pressure ventilation (PPV) with 100% oxygen—*not* on a heart rate obtained at the time of delivery.

When to Begin

Current recommendations include two indications for initiating chest compressions.

Chest compressions are indicated if *after* 15–30 seconds of PPV with 100% oxygen the heart rate is:

- **Below 60, or**
- **Between 60 and 80 and *not* increasing.**

When to Stop

Once the heart rate is 80 beats/minute or greater, chest compressions should be discontinued.

Note:

Some experienced individuals prefer to intubate an infant before or shortly after initiating chest compressions. However, chest compressions can be carried out in an infant who is being ventilated with a bag and mask. A person who is inexperienced with intubation should not take the time to attempt to intubate an asphyxiated infant who is in need of chest compressions.

Summary

The steps leading to initiating and discontinuing chest compressions are:

1. Ventilate infant with 100% oxygen for 15–30 seconds.

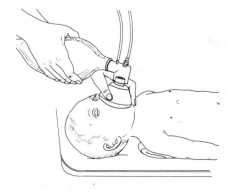

2. Evaluate heart rate.

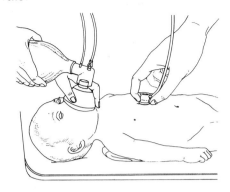

3. Initiate chest compressions if:
HR less than 60, or *between 60 and 80 and **not** increasing.*

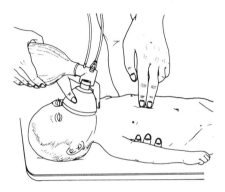

4. Reevaluate heart rate:
Below 80—
Continue chest
compressions.

80 or above—
Discontinue chest
compressions.

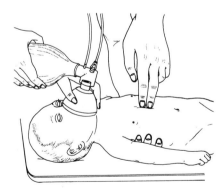 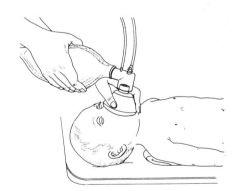

Practice Activity 1

This practice activity will help test your knowledge of some key concepts, including when to initiate chest compressions.

Fill In

1. When should chest compressions be initiated in a neonate? Include the two heart rate indications and the required ventilatory support.

   _____

   _____

   _____

2. When should chest compressions be discontinued?

   _____

3. Chest compressions must always be accompanied by _____

   _____

Case Situation

A severely asphyxiated apneic infant is delivered, requiring both ventilation and chest compressions. List in *proper sequence* what you would do for this infant. Select from the actions given. You will need to recall information learned in previous lessons in this series.

Actions

4. _____   **A.** Suction mouth and nose

5. _____   **B.** Place on a warmer

6. _____   **C.** Chest compressions

7. _____   **D.** Dry infant

8. _____   **E.** Slap foot

9. _____   **F.** Ventilate with 100% oxygen

10. _____   **G.** Hold oxygen tubing $1/2''$ from nose

11. _____   **H.** Position with neck slightly extended

   I. Obtain heart rate

Practice Activity 1: Answers

After checking your answers, be sure to review any information about which you feel uncertain.

Fill In

1. If after ventilating with 100% oxygen for 15—30 seconds the heart rate is less than 60 or between 60 and 80 beats/minute and not increasing

2. When the heart rate is 80 or above

3. Positive-pressure ventilation with 100% oxygen

Case Situation

4. B

5. D

6. H

7. A

8. E

9. F

10. I

11. C

Decision

If . . .	Then . . .
You were correct on all 11 . . .	Great. Go on to the next section of the lesson.
You missed any question . . .	Review the appropriate material before going on, as this information is essential to the procedure.

Positioning for Chest Compressions

When the decision to initiate chest compressions is made, the infant is already positioned for positive-pressure ventilation and is being ventilated with 100% oxygen. The person performing chest compressions must gain access to the chest and place his or her hands appropriately. It is important that the two people position themselves in such a way that each one can do an effective job without interfering with the other.

In this part of the lesson we will deal mainly with the technique, including the positioning of hands (and fingers or thumbs), used in compressing a neonate's chest.

Two Techniques

You will learn two different techniques that can be used in performing chest compressions. These techniques are:
- Thumb technique, and
- Two-finger technique.

Thumb Technique

With the thumb technique, the two thumbs are used to depress the sternum, with the hands encircling the torso and the fingers supporting the back.

Two-Finger Technique

With the two-finger technique, the tips of the middle finger and either the index finger or ring finger of one hand are used to compress the sternum. The other hand is used to support the infant's back, unless the infant is on a very firm surface.

These two techniques have several things in common:
- Position of the infant
  - Firm support for the back
  - Neck slightly extended
- Compressions
  - Same location, depth, and rate

It is advantageous that you learn both methods of performing chest compressions. Each method has advantages and disadvantages.

Location of Compression

When chest compressions are performed on a neonate, pressure is applied to the lower third of the sternum. Care must be used to avoid applying pressure to the xiphoid.

To locate the area, imagine a line drawn between the nipples. The lower third of the sternum is just below this line.

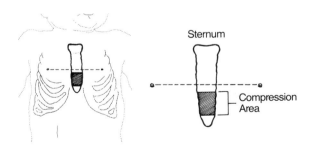

Using the Thumbs

The first technique we will discuss is the one in which the thumbs are used for compressing the sternum. This is accomplished by encircling the torso with both hands and placing the thumbs on the sternum and the fingers under the infant. The thumbs can be placed side by side or, on a small infant, one over the other.

Thumb Placement

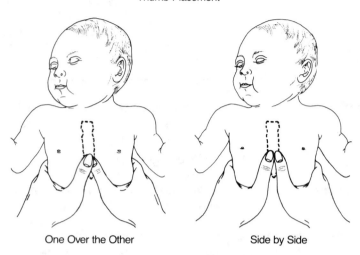

One Over the Other   Side by Side

The thumbs will be used to compress the sternum, while your fingers provide the support needed for the back. Care must be taken *not* to squeeze the chest (ribs) with your whole hand during compression. If the chest is squeezed, the infant may suffer fractured ribs or a pneumothorax.

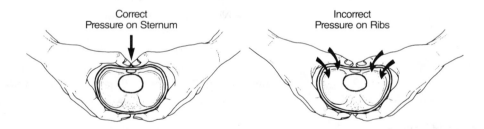

Correct
Pressure on Sternum   Incorrect
Pressure on Ribs

Note:

The thumb technique has some restrictions. It cannot be used effectively if the infant is large or your hands are small. It also makes access to the umbilical cord more difficult when medications become necessary. However, you will find the thumb technique less tiresome than the two-finger technique if chest compressions are required for a prolonged period of time.

Practice

Using your manikin, position your hands as described for this technique.
- Are your thumbs below an imaginary line drawn between the nipples?
- Are your hands large enough so that pressure will not be applied to the ribs as you compress the heart?

Two-Finger Method

In the second technique, the tips of your middle finger and either the index or ring finger of one hand are used for compression. You will probably find it easier to use your right hand if you are right-handed, the left if you are left-handed. Position the two fingers perpendicular to the chest as shown below, and press with your fingertips. If you find that your nails prevent you from using your fingertips, you should ventilate the infant while your partner compresses the chest. Or, you could use the thumb method for performing chest compressions.

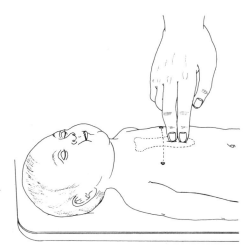

When compressing the chest, only the two fingertips should rest on the chest. In this way, you can best control the pressure you apply to the sternum. If you rest other portions of your hand on the chest, you can restrict chest expansion during ventilation, and you can apply pressure to vulnerable areas of the chest, risking a pneumothorax or fractured ribs.

Chest Compression

Correct

Incorrect

Your other hand can be used to support the infant's back so that the heart is more effectively compressed between the sternum and spine. (If the infant is positioned on a very firm surface, this may not be necessary.) With the second hand supporting the back, you can feel the pressure and the depth of compressions.

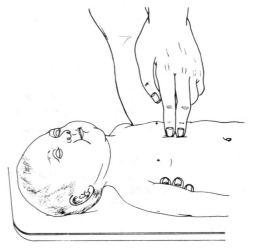

Note:

This technique is more tiring than the thumb technique if chest compressions are required for a prolonged period of time. However, the two-finger method can be used regardless of the size of the infant or the size of your hands. An additional advantage of this technique is that it leaves the umbilicus free, in case medications need to be administered via the umbilical route.

Practice

Using your manikin, position your hands and fingers appropriately for the two-finger method.

- Is one hand under the infant to provide a firm surface?
- Are two fingertips of the other hand placed vertically on the sternum, just below an imaginary line drawn between the nipples?
- Are the two fingers perpendicular to the sternum?

Position of the Infant

Remember that an infant who is being ventilated and whose chest is being compressed must be properly positioned for both procedures. The infant's neck must be slightly extended to provide an open airway for ventilation.

Thumb method: Use your fingers to support the infant's back, and use both thumbs to compress the sternum.

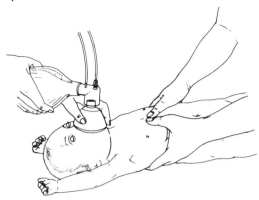

Two-finger method: Use the tips of two fingers of one hand to compress the sternum, and use your other hand or a very firm surface to support the infant's back.

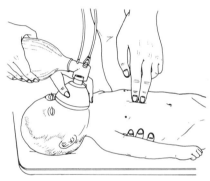

Position of Resuscitators

In addition to positioning the infant properly, the persons providing ventilation and chest compressions must position themselves so that each can do an effective job without restricting the other.

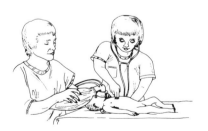

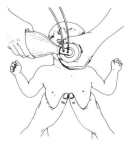

Practice Activity 2

This practice activity will help you evaluate your knowledge of key concepts. Follow the directions for each part.

Identify

1. In the diagram below, shade the area to be compressed during chest compressions on a newborn infant.

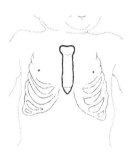

True/False

2. _____ With newborn infants, firm support for the back is not required to perform effective chest compressions.

3. _____ The nipple line of the infant crosses the center of the lower third of the sternum.

4. _____ When chest compressions are begun, ventilation with 100% oxygen should be discontinued.

5. _____ During chest compressions, care must be taken not to squeeze the chest (ribs).

6. _____ When providing chest compressions, the thumb method is generally more tiresome than the two-finger method.

7. _____ An infant receiving chest compressions and positive-pressure ventilation at the same time must be properly positioned for both procedures.

8. _____ The two-finger technique can be used on any infant, regardless of the size of the infant or the size of your hands.

Practice Activity 2: Answers

Use the following answers to check the accuracy of your responses; then review any points you may have missed.

Identify

1.

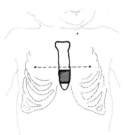

Compression Area
(lower third of sternum — area just below a line drawn between the nipples)

True/False

2. **False** — Even in neonates, firm support for the back is important. This can be provided by either a very firm surface or your fingers or hand.

3. **False** — The lower third of the sternum falls just below a line drawn between the nipples.

4. **False** — It is essential that ventilation with 100% oxygen is continued so that the blood circulated by means of the chest compressions will be oxygenated.

5. **True**

6. **False** — It is *less* tiresome over long periods.

7. **True**

8. **True**

Decision

If . . .	Then . . .
You had at least 7 of the 8 items correct . . .	Good work! Review any points about which you had some question, then continue.
You missed 2 or more answers . . .	Take time to review this section before you move on.

Compression

Thus far, you have learned to position the infant for both chest compressions and ventilation, locate the correct area of the sternum, and position hands and fingers or thumbs for performing chest compressions. Now let's look at some details about compressing the sternum. In this section, we will illustrate the two-finger method of compression.

Pressure

Controlling the pressure used in compressing the sternum is an important part of the procedure.

With your fingers and hands correctly positioned, you should use enough pressure to depress the sternum *1/2 to 3/4 inch,* then release the pressure to allow the heart to refill. One compression consists of the downward stroke plus the release.

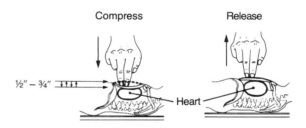

Practice

On the manikin, practice compressing the sternum 1/2 to 3/4 inch, using each of the two techniques.

Rate

The *rate* at which you compress is also very important. Remember that chest compressions take the place of the normal function of the heart, so your goal is to carry on the compressions at a rate that is close to the normal heart rate of a neonate. This means that you should repeat the compression/release action *120 times per minute.* If this rate seems high, remember that neonates normally have a faster heart rate than adults, so chest compressions on infants must be performed at a faster rate.

Practice

To become familiar with how rapidly you must compress the chest in a neonate, practice by mimicking the movements or tapping a table top at a rate of 120 times per minute. In doing so, you should be compressing your fingers or tapping at a rate of 10 for each 5 seconds (2 per second). It is important to have a feeling for this rate before proceeding to learn the actual procedure.

Do Not Remove Thumbs or Fingers from the Chest

Your thumbs or the tips of your fingers (depending on the method you are using) should remain in contact with the compression area of the sternum at all times, during both compression *and* release. *Do not* lift your thumbs or fingers off the chest between compressions.

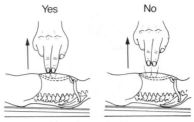

Yes   No

Remain in Contact with Chest
at Release

If you take your fingers or thumbs completely off the sternum after compression:

- You waste time relocating the compression area.
- You lose control over the depth of compression.
- You may compress the wrong area, producing trauma to the chest or underlying organs.

Be Consistent

It is very important that you keep both the *depth* and the *rate* of the compressions consistent. To assure adequate circulation, the compressions should be delivered at a steady rate and a consistent depth. *Keep the depth of the compressions at approximately 1/2 to 3/4 inch and the rate at approximately 120 per minute.*

Note:

When you are performing chest compressions on an infant, you are the "pump" for the infant's heart, and the circulation depends on your chest compressions. Any interruption in compressions will result in a precipitous drop in blood pressure as circulation ceases. Therefore, it is important to be consistent in the compression rate.

Practice

Before going on, stop to practice chest compressions on a manikin. Keep in mind the important principles. Are you:

- Compressing 1/2 to 3/4 inch?
- At a rate of 120/minute (10 in 5 seconds)?
- Compressing the sternum — not ribs (thumb method)?
- Keeping your fingers perpendicular (two-finger method)?
- Not lifting your fingers or thumbs off the chest?
- Steady in the rate and depth of compressions?

Checking Effectiveness

It is important to know whether the blood is being circulated effectively as a result of the chest compressions. To determine this, the pulse should be checked periodically, if at all possible. It would be very helpful to have a third person readily available to do this.

Practice

When in the nursery, practice palpating the various pulses of a neonate, e.g., carotid, brachial, and femoral. Which is easiest for you to detect? You must be confident in your ability to palpate pulses on a normal neonate before trying to do so on an infant with compromised cardiac output.

Anatomy and Dangers Related to Chest Compressions

Chest compressions can cause trauma to the infant. To help minimize complications as chest compressions are performed, information on the anatomy of the chest is presented below. The vital organs that lie within the rib cage are also identified. Finally, the complications that can result from chest compressions are discussed.

Location of Organs

Two vital organs lie within the rib cage: the heart and lungs. In addition, the liver lies partially under the ribs, although it is in the abdominal cavity.

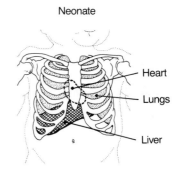

Neonate

Heart

Lungs

Liver

Dangers

As you perform chest compressions, you must apply enough pressure to compress the heart between the sternum and spine, without damaging underlying organs.

Broken Ribs

The ribs are fragile and can easily be broken. The splintered edges can then puncture underlying organs and cause hemorrhage or a pneumothorax.

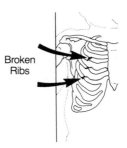

Broken Ribs

Lacerated Liver

The lower tip of the sternum, called the *xiphoid process,* is spear-shaped and curves inward. Pressure over the xiphoid can lead to laceration of the liver.

Pneumothorax

Trauma to the rib cage during compressions can cause a pneumothorax.
By following the procedure outlined in this lesson, the above injuries can be minimized.

Practice Activity 3

Complete the items given below, using the information you have just finished reading.

Fill In

1. What depth should you use when you compress the infant's sternum?

   _____

2. Chest compressions should be performed on a neonate at the rate of _____ times per minute.

3–4. What two vital organs lie within the rib cage?

   • _____

   • _____

True/False

5. _____ The pressure used in compressing the sternum is directly related to the rate at which you deliver the compressions.

6. _____ In chest compressions, one "compression" consists of the downward stroke plus the release.

7. _____ It does not matter if you lift your thumbs (or fingers) off the infant's chest between compressions.

8. _____ You should keep both the depth and rate of the compressions consistent.

Selection

9–11. Which of the following were given as complications that can result from chest compressions? (Place an "X" in front of each correct answer.)

   A. _____ Broken ribs

   B. _____ Cardiac arrest

   C. _____ Lacerated liver

   D. _____ Pneumothorax

   E. _____ Fractured clavicle

Multiple Choice

Select the correct answers by placing a check mark (✔) in front of the appropriate statements.

12–14. Regardless of the method used, problems can occur if you take your thumbs or fingers completely off the sternum between compressions. In the list given below, check the statements that indicate what might happen.

   A. _____ You lose control over the depth of compression.

   B. _____ You may decrease the concentration of oxygen delivered to the infant.

   C. _____ You may compress the wrong area, producing trauma.

   D. _____ You waste time relocating the compression area.

Practice Activity 3: Answers

Carefully compare your responses to the ones given below.

Fill In

1. $1/2$ to $3/4$ inch

2. 120 times per minute

3–4. • Heart
      • Lungs

True/False

5. **False** — Pressure is dependent upon the *depth* to which you compress the sternum, not the rate.

6. **True**

7. **False** — Your thumbs (or the tips of your fingers) should remain in contact with the lower third of the sternum at all times, during compression *and* release.

8. **True**

Selection

9–11. **A, C, D**

Multiple Choice

12–14. **A, C, D**

Decision

If . . .	Then . . .
Your score was 13 or more . . .	You are doing well! Go right on to the section entitled "Ventilation During Chest Compressions."
You had a score of *less* than 13 . . .	You should look again at the material that deals with the items you missed. Then retake the practice activity before you go on.

Ventilation During Chest Compressions

During cardiopulmonary resuscitation, positive-pressure ventilation *must* always accompany chest compressions. It has previously been suggested that the two procedures be coordinated so that ventilations do not occur when the chest is compressed. There are currently no data for the intubated neonate to suggest that interposed ventilations have either an advantage or disadvantage over simultaneous ventilations and chest compressions.

Air in Stomach

When performing bag-mask ventilation with simultaneous chest compressions, an occasional intermittent breath will be given at the same time the chest is compressed. In these circumstances, gas will follow a path of least resistance and is more likely to enter the stomach. When ventilating with a bag and mask during chest compressions, interposing a breath between every third compression may have some advantages. Whether or not ventilations are interposed with compressions, an orogastric tube should be used to decompress the stomach when bag-mask ventilation is prolonged or there is evidence of gastric distension. An endotracheal tube may be the best way to provide ventilation during simultaneous chest compressions, particularly if the need for chest compressions is prolonged.

Ventilation Rate

During chest compressions, positive-pressure ventilations with 100% oxygen should be performed *at a rate of 40–60/minute.*

Evaluation of Heart Rate

Remember that chest compressions should be instituted if, **after 15—30 seconds of positive-pressure ventilation with 100% oxygen**, the heart rate is:
- Below 60 or
- Between 60 and 80 and **not** increasing

Chest compressions should be **stopped** when the heart rate reaches **80 beats/minute or greater**.

Checking Heart Rate

During chest compressions, the infant's heart rate should be checked frequently to determine whether chest compressions should be continued.

Initially

After an initial 30 seconds of chest compressions, the heart rate should be checked.

Later

The infant's heart rate should be checked periodically when chest compressions are being performed. In an infant showing a positive response to chest compressions, the heart rate should be checked as frequently as every 30 seconds so that you can discontinue compressions as soon as the heart rate is 80 per minute or above. Heart-rate checks may be performed at less frequent intervals in infants requiring prolonged cardiopulmonary resuscitation.

6-Second Heart Rate

The heart rate should be checked for no longer than 6 seconds. The 6-second heart rate gives you the needed information with a minimal interruption in chest compressions.

Note:

If a stethoscope is used, ventilation should be discontinued while the heart rate is checked so that breath sounds do not obscure the heart beat.

Evaluating the Heart Rate

Below 80 (Continue)

A heart rate of less than 80 per minute indicates that the infant has inadequate circulation to the vital organs. Chest compressions and ventilation must continue.

Such an infant may also be intubated and may be receiving biochemical resuscitation.

As long as the infant does not have a spontaneous heart rate of 80 or above, chest compressions should continue. The decision to cease cardiopulmonary resuscitation in an infant who does not have a spontaneous heart rate is a medical one and depends on an assessment of the cerebral and cardiovascular status.

80 or Above (Discontinue)

A heart rate of 80 beats/minute or above indicates that compressions should be discontinued. Ventilation should be continued until the heart rate is above 100 and the infant is capable of breathing spontaneously.

Decision

- Heart rate of less than 80:
    - Continue chest compressions.
    - Continue ventilation with 100% oxygen.
    - Continue to check heart rate periodically.
    - Initiate medications.

- Heart rate of 80 or above:
    - Discontinue chest compressions.
    - Continue ventilation until heart rate is above 100 and infant is breathing spontaneously.

Practice Activity 4

This practice activity provides a means of evaluating your knowledge of key concepts from the two previous sections of this lesson.

Fill In

1. In an infant receiving chest compressions, ventilations should be administered at a rate of _____–_____/minute.

2. How long after initiating chest compressions should you continue before checking the heart rate? _____

True/False

3. _____ Because of the infant's critical condition, the heart rate should be checked for no longer than 30 seconds.

4. _____ As long as an infant does not have a spontaneous heart rate of 80 or above, chest compressions should continue.

5. _____ Anytime an infant being given chest compressions achieves an adequate spontaneous heart rate, it is safe to discontinue *both* the ventilations and the chest compressions.

6. _____ A heart rate of 60–80 or below indicates that the circulation of blood to the vital organs is inadequate.

Practice Activity 4: Answers

As you check your answers for this practice activity, review the content for any items you missed or about which you have some uncertainty.

Fill In

1. 40–60/minute

2. 30 seconds

True/False

3. False — The heart rate should be checked for no more than *6* seconds. Using the 6-second heart rate keeps the interruption in chest compressions at a minimum.

4. True

5. False — Ventilations should continue if the infant is not yet breathing on his or her own, or if the heart rate is below 100.

6. True

Decision

If . . .	**Then . . .**
You had 5 or 6 items correct . . .	You are doing well. Go right on to the "Review of the Procedure."
You missed more than 1 of the answers . . .	Before you turn to the "Review of the Procedure," go back to the content given in the preceding two sections and make sure that you understand and can remember each of the points presented.

Review of the Procedure

This is a review of the order in which the steps are carried out in the chest-compression procedure.

Indications for Chest Compressions

The infant in need of chest compressions has:

- A heart rate below 60, or between 60 and 80 and not increasing, after 15–30 seconds of ventilation with 100% oxygen.

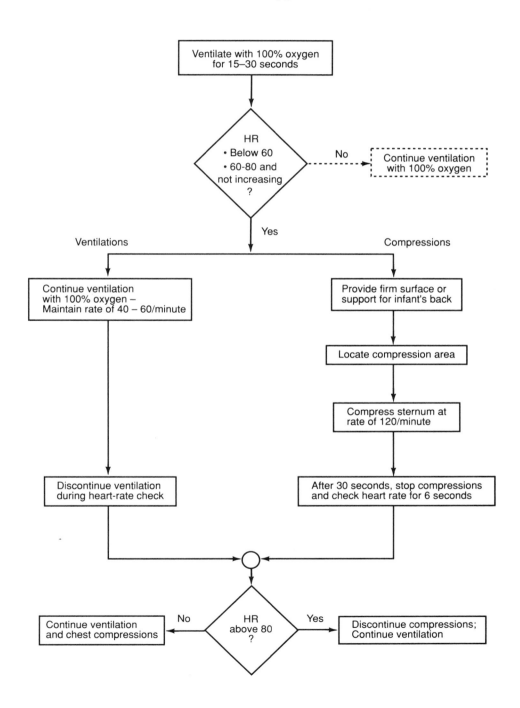

Case Study

Here is a case study of an infant from the identification of apnea through chest compressions. The timing of the procedure is given at the left, so you will see how quickly these actions take place.

Time: 0:00
(min:sec)
Position and Suction

An infant has just been delivered and is apneic. You quickly place him under a heated warmer and dry his entire body. You position him and suction the mouth and nose. As you observe the chest, there is no respiratory effort. You provide tactile stimulation.

Time: 0:20
Ventilate

As there still is no respiratory effort, you immediately ventilate with a bag and mask, using 100% oxygen. After attaining and checking the seal between the mask and the infant's face, you ventilate the infant for 15–30 seconds, maintaining a rate of 40–60 per minute.

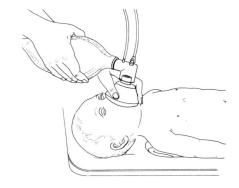

Next, you check the heart rate for 6 seconds, and detect 3 beats. That means the rate is below 60 per minute. With a heart rate that slow, chest compressions must be initiated.

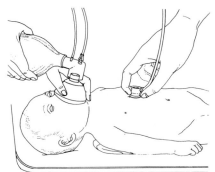

Time: 0:55
Prepare for Chest Compressions

Time: 1:10

Alert a second person to initiate chest compressions while you continue ventilation, or have someone else ventilate the infant and you initiate compressions.

While your coworker takes over ventilation, you position one hand under the infant's back and position your fingertips on the sternum, just *below* an imaginary line drawn between the nipples. (Or, use both hands to encircle the chest, with the thumbs compressing the sternum and the fingertips supporting the back.)

Provide Chest Compressions

You begin chest compressions at a rate of 120 per minute.

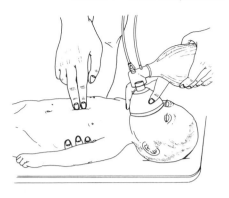

Check Heart Rate

After 30 seconds of chest compressions and ventilation, you check the heart rate. Your coworker ceases ventilation so that you can listen carefully for 6 seconds. You detect 5 beats, which is well below 80 per minute. Continued chest compressions are needed.

Time: 1:50

Continue

Ventilations are resumed, and you quickly relocate the compression area and begin again. After another 30 seconds have elapsed, you check the heart rate again.

Time: 2:20

Improvement

This time the heart rate is up to 90. With the heart rate above 80 per minute, chest compressions are no longer necessary, but ventilation with 100% oxygen is continued. You announce the heart rate.

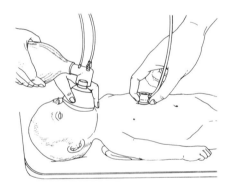

You check the heart rate periodically over the next 2 minutes, and it slowly increases to 140.

Time: 4:25

End

The resuscitation team continues to ventilate the infant. Once spontaneous respirations are evident, ventilation will be discontinued. Should the infant's heart rate again drop to below 80 per minute, chest compressions must be resumed.

Summary

This is a brief review of the information about chest compressions. Study this carefully before taking the posttest.

Heart Rate

The decision to initiate chest compressions is based on the neonate's heart rate. The condition under which chest compressions are necessary is:

Heart rate below 60, or between 60 and 80 and *not* increasing, despite 15–30 seconds of ventilation with 100% oxygen.

Position Infant

The infant is already in position for ventilation with the neck slightly extended. You must provide firm support for the back so that the heart can be compressed between the sternum and the spine.

If the infant's back is firmly supported, you are ready to begin chest compressions.

If the back is not firmly supported and you are using the two-finger method, place one hand under the infant's back.

If using the thumb method, quickly encircle the torso with your hands.

Position Fingers or Thumbs

While another person continues ventilations, quickly locate the lower third of the sternum and position your fingertips or thumbs as shown below.

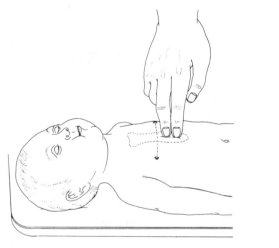 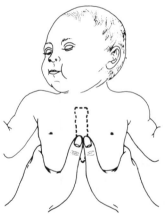

Two-Finger Method: The tips of the middle and index or ring finger should be used for compression.

Thumb Method: The balls of the thumbs should be used for compression.

Rates

The sternum should be compressed at the rate of 120 times per minute, to a depth of $1/2$ to $3/4$ inch. Ventilation should occur at a rate of 40–60/minute.

Check Heart

After 30 seconds of compressions and ventilations, check the heart rate for 6 seconds. If the heart rate is:

- **Below 80 per minute**—continue compressions and ventilation.

- **80 per minute or greater**—discontinue compressions, but continue ventilation with 100% oxygen.

Remember, even if the heart rate is found to be zero, compressions and ventilation should continue until a medical decision is reached to discontinue resuscitation.

Practice

You are now ready to practice combining chest compressions and ventilations. To practice this procedure, you must work with either an instructor or a coworker who has completed the lessons on bag and mask and chest compressions.

1. Practice both methods of chest compressions.

2. Practice ventilating while the other person provides chest compressions.

Suggestion: Place your manikin on a radiant warmer for practice. Performing chest compressions and ventilation at the height of the warmer is quite different from doing it on a table top. Practicing with the manikin on a warmer will help you feel comfortable with your position and that of the infant. Remember, in a real situation, cardiopulmonary resuscitation is performed on a warming table.

Use the performance checklist at the end of this lesson to determine if you are performing correctly and if you are ready for clinical testing.

Posttest
Lesson 4 — Chest Compressions

Name _____ Date _____

Before you go on to the clinical practice portion of this lesson, here is a chance to test yourself on the key concepts and facts about chest compressions. Follow the directions for each section.

Identify

1. Shade the area of the infant's chest that should be compressed when performing chest compressions.

Fill In

For the following questions, fill in the blank with the appropriate word or phrase.

2. When should chest compressions be initiated in a neonate? Include the two heart-rate indications and the required ventilatory support.

   _____

   _____

   _____

3. Chest compressions should always be accompanied by

   _____.

   What part(s) of the hand should be used when compressing the neonate's sternum?

4. Thumb Method: _____

5. Two-Finger Method: _____

6. Chest compressions should be performed on a neonate at the rate of _____ per minute.

7. During chest compressions, ventilations should be administered at a rate of _____–_____ per minute.

8–9. List at least two complications that can result from chest compressions.

* _____

* _____

10. At what heart rate should chest compressions be discontinued?

_____ per minute.

11. After initiating chest compressions, how long should you continue before checking the heart rate?

_____

12. If you were the person *ventilating* an infant who is receiving chest compressions, what should you do while your co-worker checks the baby's heart rate with a stethoscope?

_____

If you were doing the *chest compressions* on an infant, would you continue or discontinue *compressions* in infants with the following 6-second heart rates?

6-second H.R.

13.   9   _____

14.   6   _____

15.   12   _____

As the person *ventilating* an infant who is receiving chest compressions, would you continue or discontinue *ventilation* in infants with the following heart rates?

H.R.

16.   90   _____

17.   70   _____

18.   130   _____

Lesson 4 Posttest: Answers

Check your answers with those given here.

Identify

1.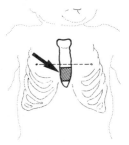

Compression Area
(lower third of sternum — area below a line drawn between the nipples and above the xiphoid)

Fill In

2. If despite ventilation with 100% oxygen for 15–30 seconds the heart rate is less than 60, or is between 60 and 80 beats per minute and not increasing

3. Positive-pressure ventilation with 100% oxygen

4. Thumbs of both hands

5. Fingertips of middle and either index or ring finger

6. 120 per minute

7. 40–60 per minute

8–9. Broken ribs

   Laceration of liver

   Pneumothorax

   (Any two of the above are acceptable.)

10. 80 per minute or above

11. 30 seconds

12. Discontinue ventilation while co-worker checks H.R.

13. Discontinue chest compressions

14. Continue chest compressions

15. Discontinue chest compressions

16. Continue ventilation

17. Continue ventilation

18. Discontinue ventilation if infant has spontaneous respirations

Decision

If . . .	Then . . .
You had 16 out of 18 items correct . . .	You have mastered the information in this lesson and are ready to go through the performance checklist.
You missed more than 2 questions . . .	Review the information related to the questions you missed; then retake the posttest.

Performance Checklist
Lesson 4—Chest Compressions

Instructions

Instructor: This checklist has two parts: one for judging compression and one for judging ventilation. The participant should be instructed to talk through the procedure as it is demonstrated. Judge the performance of each step. Check (✔) when the action is completed correctly. If done incorrectly, circle the box so that you can discuss that step later.

The demonstration should be done on an infant resuscitation manikin. Where you see two stars (**) you are to provide information regarding the "infant's" condition. This allows you to check the participant's ability to make the correct decision and take appropriate actions based on that decision. Since time is of the essence in resuscitation, you will find a space for rating the overall speed of the demonstration. The participant should be able to carry out the steps and make the correct decisions at approximately the same rate as in an actual resuscitation.

Chest compressions must be demonstrated while ventilations are coordinated with the compressions. For the first part of the checklist the instructor, or someone who has completed the lesson, ventilates while the participant compresses. For the second part the roles are reversed. The participant must be taken through the "Compression" part of the checklist twice in order to demonstrate both methods of performing chest compressions.

Equipment and Supplies

Infant resuscitation manikin
Resuscitation bag and mask
Pressure gauge, if used
Oxygen reservoir, if using a self-inflating bag
Oxygen equipment
    Oxygen source
    Flowmeter
    Oxygen tubing
    Air/oxygen blender, if used
Stethoscope
20-cc syringe, 8 Fr. feeding tube, 1/2" x 2" piece of adhesive tape
Clock with a second hand
Bulb syringe
Shoulder roll
Blanket for drying infant

Performance Checklist
Lesson 4 — Chest Compressions

Name _____ Instructor _____ Date _____

Compression

Situation:

"This baby has been ventilated with 100% oxygen for 30 seconds. I've checked the heart rate, and I detected 5 beats in 6 seconds. I am going to continue to ventilate while you get ready. You take charge of the situation now."

Positions fingers or thumbs on chest

☐ **1A. Two-finger method**
Places fingertips of middle and index or ring finger immediately below a line between the nipples and above the xiphoid process

☐ **1B. Thumb method**
Places balls of thumbs immediately below a line between the nipples and above the xiphoid process

☐ **2. Provides a firm support for infant's back**

☐ **3. Brings tempo to approximately 120 compressions per minute within 10–15 seconds**

☐ **4. Maintains tempo at 120 thereafter**

☐ **5. Compresses sternum 1/2 to 3/4 inch**

☐ **6. Keeps fingertips/thumbs on sternum during release**

☐ **7. Checks heart rate after 30 seconds of compressions**

☐ **8. Checks heart rate for exactly 6 seconds**

**Instructor: Choose one of the situations below.

"You detect 6 beats."

"You detect 9 beats."

☐ **9A. Repositions fingers and resumes chest compressions**

☐ **9B. Discontinues chest compressions while ventilation continues**

Ventilation

Situation:

"This infant has been dried, positioned, suctioned, and given tactile stimulation, but remains apneic. You take charge of the situation. I'm available to offer assistance if requested."

↓

☐ **1. Initiates bag-and-mask ventilation with 100% oxygen**

↓

☐ **2. After 15–30 seconds of ventilation the participant checks the heart rate or asks you to do so**

↓

**Instructor: "The heart rate is 4 in 6 seconds."

↓

☐ **3. Participant indicates infant needs chest compressions**

↓

☐ **4. With a second person performing chest compressions, the participant continues ventilating at a rate of 40–60 per minute**

↓

☐ **5. Provides adequate ventilation pressure**

↓

☐ **6. After 30 seconds of chest compressions, states heart rate should be taken**

↓

☐ **7. Ceases ventilation while second person checks heart rate**

↓

☐ **8. Resumes ventilation immediately after heart rate check**

↓

☐ **9. Correctly states whether chest compressions should be stopped or continued, depending on heart rate**

Overall

☐ Speed—carried out actions without undue delays

☐ Correctly performed two-finger method

☐ Correctly performed thumb method

Endotracheal Intubation   Lesson 5

Contents

Endotracheal Intubation

Lesson 5

Introduction to Lesson 5

Endotracheal intubation is perhaps the most difficult skill to *maintain* of those taught in the *Textbook of Neonatal Resuscitation*. Even though one may initially master the skill, if it is not practiced regularly, one can "lose the touch" rather easily.

This lesson teaches the concepts and basic skills of endotracheal intubation. Additional supervised experience is required to assume clinical responsibility for endotracheal intubation. That additional experience required before assuming clinical responsibilities will depend on guidelines established by the hospital.

In addition to teaching endotracheal intubation of a neonate, this lesson has been designed to teach the information and skills necessary for staff who assist with the procedure.

Two Roles

It is possible for an unassisted, skilled operator to perform endotracheal intubation on a neonate. However, the assistance of a second person— knowledgeable about the equipment required and the steps in the procedure— can be instrumental in assuring that the procedure is carried out quickly and with a greater likelihood of success. During most of the procedure, the operator must have a laryngoscope in one hand, ET tube or suction catheter in the other, and eyes fixed on the glottis. The assistant is left to anticipate what is needed, offer equipment when appropriate, and monitor the infant's response to the procedure.

This lesson has been written to provide both the operator and assistant with the knowledge and skills each will need in performing his or her particular role.

Overview of the Lesson

This lesson has two major sections. One describes the flow of the procedure, and the other is a guide for practicing intubation.

The first section contains:

• Discussion of the indications for endotracheal intubation,

• List of the equipment required,

• Detailed description of the procedure, and

• Posttest.

The last part of the lesson contains an outline for guided practice in developing the manual skills involved in performing intubation. It is designed to be used with an infant intubation manikin.

What to Study

Both the operator and assistant should complete the entire first part of the lesson up through the posttest. The practice guide, which follows the posttest, was specifically designed for the operator. However, those assisting with intubation may choose to go through it to become more familiar with the intubation procedure.

The lesson contains two performance checklists—one for the individual assisting and another for the operator.

If you have any questions about your responsibilities in the intubation procedure, discuss them with your supervisor.

Prerequisites

Before you attempt this lesson, the other resuscitation procedures should be thoroughly understood. These include:
- The initial steps of resuscitation—including positioning, suctioning, and tactile stimulation,
- Ventilation using a resuscitation bag and mask, and
- Chest compressions.

Objectives

To successfully complete the *knowledge* portion of this lesson, you must be able to:

Knowledge

- Know the indications for performing endotracheal intubation on a neonate.
- State the steps in:
  - Preparing an ET tube,
  - Inserting the laryngoscope and ET tube,
  - Preventing or minimizing hypoxia, and
  - Initial and final confirmation of tube placement.
- Select from a series of illustrations:
  - Correct positions of the infant for endotracheal intubation, and
  - Correct positioning of the laryngoscope.
- Label on a diagram:
  - Esophagus, epiglottis, glottis, vallecula, vocal cords, trachea, carina, and mainstem bronchi, and
  - Three places you would listen for air entry when checking ET tube placement.
- When given the weight of an infant, state the correct size of endotracheal tube to be used.
- State the suction pressure appropriate for suctioning a neonate.
- Identify correct statements related to the intubation procedure.
- State the maximum time allowed for each intubation attempt.
- Given specific signs related to placement of the ET tube, correctly state where the tip of the tube is positioned; and if incorrectly positioned, state the corrective measure that should be taken.
- List four complications that can result from intubation.

Operator Performance

To complete the *clinical* portion of this lesson, the operator must be able to:

- Perform endotracheal intubation on an infant intubation manikin or an appropriately anesthetized animal model.

Performance will be judged using the performance checklist on page 5-72, entitled "Performing Endotracheal Intubation."

Note:

American Heart Association policy is that the acquisition, care, and use of animals by the personnel and the institution involved in this course must conform to the guidelines set forth in the National Institutes of Health's *Public Health Service Policy on Humane Care and Use of Laboratory Animals.* An absolute corollary is that the instructional session in which the use of animals is contemplated must be held in a facility that is licensed by the Public Health Service for compliance with the policy.

Assistant Performance

The assistant must be able to:

Prepare the supplies and equipment needed for intubating a neonate.

Demonstrate on an infant manikin (not an intubation head) the following:
• Correct position of infant for intubation,
• Application of pressure over the trachea,
• Procedure for providing free-flow oxygen,
• Steps for initially confirming tube placement, and
• Securing tube to face.

Performance will be judged using the performance checklist on page 5-68, entitled "Assisting with Intubation."

Decision Table

If . . .	Then . . .
You feel you can pass a test on these objectives . . .	Turn to the posttest on page 5-53.
You wish to know more before attempting the test . . .	Continue on the next page.

Indications for Endotracheal Intubation

When positive-pressure ventilation (PPV) is required on a newborn, it can be delivered with a resuscitation bag and mask or a bag and endotracheal tube. An advantage of the bag and mask is that ventilation can be initiated immediately, without the delay necessitated by the insertion of an endotracheal tube.

Endotracheal intubation is necessary in the following four situations:

• When prolonged positive-pressure ventilation is required.
• When bag-and-mask ventilation is ineffective.
• When tracheal suctioning is required.
• When diaphragmatic hernia is suspected.

Prolonged PPV Required: A bag and mask can be used to ventilate the neonate effectively over a period of time. However, when prolonged assisted ventilation is anticipated, it is easier if the infant is intubated.

Bag and Mask Ineffective: If bag-and-mask ventilation is ineffective, as evidenced by inadequate chest expansion or continuing low heart rate, the infant should be intubated.

Tracheal Suctioning: Intubation is required in order to suction the trachea of an infant born with thick or particulate meconium in the amniotic fluid. Tracheal suctioning is also indicated in infants suspected of having aspirated formula or other foreign material.

Diaphragmatic Hernia Suspected: If a diaphragmatic hernia is suspected and ventilation is required, an ET tube rather than a mask should be used. This will prevent air from entering the bowel and compromising lung expansion.

Supplies and Equipment

The supplies and equipment necessary to perform endotracheal intubation should be kept together on either a resuscitation cart or intubation tray. Each delivery room, nursery, and emergency room should have a complete set of the items listed below.

Supplies and Equipment

The supplies and equipment essential for intubating a neonate include:
- Laryngoscope with an extra set of batteries and extra bulb
- Blades: Size 1 (fullterm infant)
  Size 0 (preterm infant)
  (Straight rather than curved blades are preferred for optimal visualization.)
- Endotracheal tubes with an internal diameter (ID) of 2.5 mm, 3.0 mm, 3.5 mm, and 4.0 mm
- Stylet
- Suctioning device, or suction setup with 10 Fr. suction catheter or larger
- Shoulder roll
- Roll of ½- or ¾-inch adhesive tape
- Scissors
- Oxygen tubing
- Resuscitation bag and mask capable of providing a high concentration of oxygen

Intubation Equipment

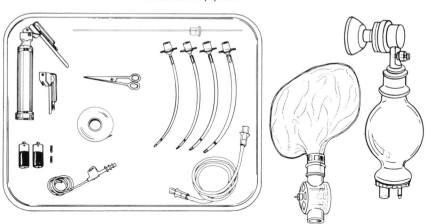

Preventing Contamination

Intubation is performed as a clean procedure; the laryngoscope blades, endotracheal tubes, and stylet should be sterile and protected from contamination. The laryngoscope handle should be thoroughly cleaned following each use.

Endotracheal Tubes

Sterile disposable tubes of nonirritating material should be used. They should be of uniform diameter throughout the length of the tube—not tapered near the tip.

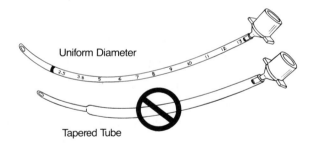

One disadvantage of the tapered tube is that during intubation, your view of the tracheal opening is easily obstructed by the wide part of the tube.

Vocal Cord Guide

Most endotracheal tubes currently manufactured for neonates have a black line near the tip of the tube, which is called a "vocal cord guide." Such tubes are meant to be inserted so that the vocal cord guide is placed at the level of the vocal cords. This usually positions the tip of the tube above the bifurcation of the trachea.

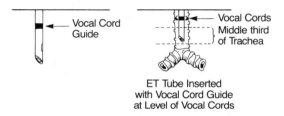

The length of the trachea in a premature infant is less than that of a fullterm infant—3 cm vs. 5–6 cm. Therefore, the smaller the tube, the closer the vocal cord guide is to the tip of the tube.

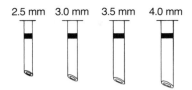

Centimeter Markings   Endotracheal tubes made for neonates come with centimeter markings along the tube, identifying the distance from the tip of the tube.

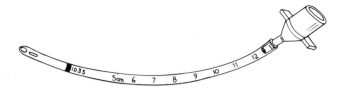

When the tube is first inserted, take note of the centimeter marking that appears at the upper lip. This can serve to alert you if the tube's position has changed.

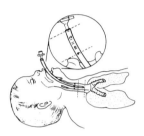

Preparing the Supplies and Equipment

Very little preparation of the supplies and equipment is necessary, once all the items are at hand. The few essential preparatory steps are discussed below:

- Selecting and preparing the endotracheal tube,
- Preparing the laryngoscope, and
- Miscellaneous preparations (tape, suction, oxygen, and bag and mask).

Selecting ET Tube

The approximate size of the endotracheal tube is determined from the infant's weight. Since preparation of equipment *prior* to a high-risk delivery is important, the chart below includes the size of tube for various gestational ages as well as for various weight categories.

Study the chart: later you will be asked to recall the suggested tube size for infants of various weights.

Tube Size (ID mm)	Weight	Gestational Age
2.5	Below 1000 gm	Below 28 weeks
3.0	1000–2000 gm	28–34 weeks
3.5	2000–3000 gm	34–38 weeks
3.5—4.0	Above 3000 gm	Above 38 weeks

Preparing ET Tube

Once you have selected the correct size tube, you will need to take several steps to prepare it for use. These include:

- Shortening the tube,
- Replacing the ET tube connector, and
- Inserting a stylet in the tube to make the tube more rigid (optional).

Shorten Tube

The ET tube can be shortened to 13 cm to make it easier to handle during intubation and to lessen the chance of inserting the tube too far. A 13 cm tube will provide enough tube to extend beyond the infant's lips for you to adjust the depth of insertion if necessary and to properly secure the tube to the face.

Cut Tube at 13 cm

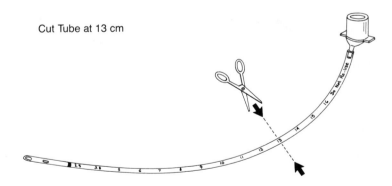

Following intubation, if more than 4 cm extends from the lips (as it will in a very small infant), the tube can easily be shortened again.

Replace Connector

After cutting the tube, replace the ET tube connector. The fitting should be tight so the connector does not inadvertently separate during insertion.

Note:

Connectors are made to fit a specific size tube. They cannot be interchanged between tubes of different sizes.

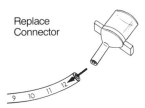

Replace Connector

Insert Stylet (Optional)

The last step in preparing an ET tube involves inserting a stylet to provide rigidity and curvature to the tube, thus facilitating intubation. When inserting the stylet, it is essential that:
- The tip does not protrude from the end of the ET tube (to prevent trauma to the tissues).
- The stylet should be secured so that it cannot advance farther into the tube during intubation.

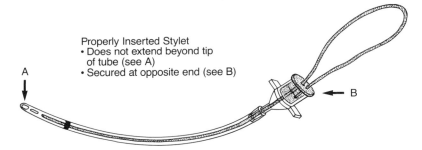

Properly Inserted Stylet
- Does not extend beyond tip of tube (see A)
- Secured at opposite end (see B)

A

B

Although many find the stylet helpful, others find the stiffness of the tube alone adequate. Use of a stylet is optional and depends on the operator's preference. Although the use of a stylet is optional, throughout the remainder of this text, we will refer to its use so the learner is prepared for its possible use in the delivery room.

Preparing Laryngoscope

To prepare the laryngoscope, first select the appropriate blade and attach it to the laryngoscope handle:

No. 0 for preterm infants, and
No. 1 for fullterm infants.

Next, turn on the light to determine that the batteries and bulb are working. Check to see that the bulb is screwed in tightly to ensure that it will not flicker or fall out during the procedure.

Additional Items

The additional items that are needed are discussed below.

Tape

Cut a strip of adhesive tape for initially securing the tube to the face. (Or obtain an ET tube holder, if used by your hospital.)

Suction Equipment

Suction equipment should be available and ready for use:
- Mechanical suction and
- 10 Fr. catheter or larger

If the endotracheal tube is left in place and one needs to suction through the tube, a 5, 6, or 8 Fr. catheter can be used, depending upon the size of the ET tube.

Suction pressure should be set so that when the suction *tubing* is occluded, the negative pressure does not exceed:

100 mm Hg

4 in Hg

Oxygen

Oxygen tubing connected to a source of 100% oxygen should be available:
- To provide an oxygen-enriched environment during intubation, and
- To use with the resuscitation bag.

Resuscitation Bag *and* Mask

A resuscitation bag and mask capable of providing 90–100% oxygen should be at hand to ventilate the infant between intubation attempts or should intubation be unsuccessful.

The bag alone will be required to ventilate the infant after intubation to initially check tube placement and to provide continued ventilation if necessary.

Summary

A summary of the steps involved in preparing for endotracheal intubation is given here:

ET tube:
- Select correct size tube.
- Shorten tube to 13 cm length.
- Reinsert connector.
- Insert stylet appropriate distance (optional).

Steps in Preparing Tube

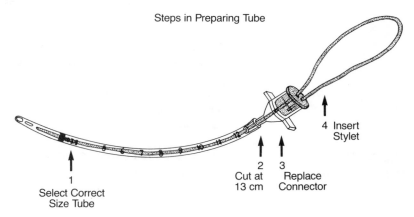

1 Select Correct Size Tube

2 Cut at 13 cm

3 Replace Connector

4 Insert Stylet

Laryngoscope:
- Attach blade, No. 0 prematures, No. 1 fullterms.
- Check light.

Additional items:
- Cut strip of tape or obtain ET tube holder.
- Prepare suction equipment.
- Prepare oxygen tube.
- Prepare resuscitation bag and mask.

Practice Activity 1

This practice activity covers the material presented so far. Follow the directions for each section.

Selection

1–4. From the following situations, select those in which endotracheal intubation is definitely indicated. _____

    A. Infants with a 1-minute Apgar score of 3 or below

    B. Infants in whom bag-and-mask fails to provide adequate ventilation

    C. Infants with thick meconium in the amniotic fluid

    D. All apneic, premature infants less than 32 weeks

    E. Infants suspected of having a diaphragmatic hernia

    F. Infants requiring prolonged positive-pressure ventilation

Completion

State the three steps involved in preparing an endotracheal tube for insertion, once a tube of the correct size has been selected.

5. _____

6. _____

7. _____

8–9. State the two steps involved in preparing a laryngoscope for use.

    • _____

    • _____

10–13. List the four additional items needed to assure that adequate equipment and supplies are available when intubating a neonate.

    • _____   • _____

    • _____   • _____

14–15. What two precautions should be taken when inserting a stylet into an ET tube to prevent complications resulting from the stylet?

    • _____

    • _____

Complete the chart below, indicating the correct ET tube size to be inserted with infants in each weight range.

Weight		Tube Size
16. Below 1000 gm	—	_____ mm
17. 1000–2000 gm	—	_____ mm
18. 2000–3000 gm	—	_____ mm
19. Above 3000 gm	—	_____ mm

20. State the suction pressure that should not be exceeded in suctioning secretions during intubation. State the pressure in terms that relate to how your gauge measures pressure. Include the correct unit of measurement (mm Hg or in Hg). _____

Practice Activity 1: Answers

Compare your answers with those given below.

Selection

1–4. B, C, E, F

Completion

5. Shorten tube to 13 cm

6. Replace ET tube connector

7. Insert stylet (optional)

8–9. • Attach correct size blade (No. 0 prematures, No. 1 fullterms)

• Check light

10–13. • Adhesive tape (or ET tube holder)

• Oxygen

• Suction equipment

• Resuscitation bag and mask

14–15. • The tip of the stylet should not extend beyond the end of the ET tube.

• The other end of the stylet should be secured so it cannot advance farther into the ET tube.

	Weight	Tube Size
16. Below 1000 gm	—	**2.5** mm
17. 1000–2000 gm	—	**3.0** mm
18. 2000–3000 gm	—	**3.5** mm
19. Above 3000 gm	—	**3.5–4.0** mm

20. 100 mm Hg
or
4 in Hg

Decision

If . . .	Then . . .
You had the correct answers to at least 19 of the 20 questions . . .	Good. Review items you may have missed; then proceed to the next page.
You missed more than 1 . . .	Reread the sections covering the questions you missed. When you are sure of the information, proceed to the next page.

Anatomy

The anatomical landmarks that relate to intubation are labelled in the illustrations below. Study the relative position of these landmarks because each is important to your understanding of the procedure.

Structures

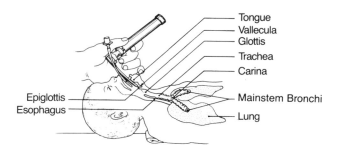

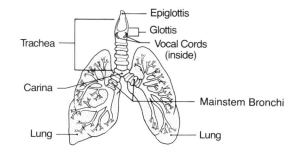

Definitions

Carina — Where the mainstem bronchi and trachea meet.

Epiglottis — A lid-like structure overhanging the entrance to the trachea.

Esophagus — The passageway extending from the throat to the stomach.

Glottis — The opening to the trachea. Contains the vocal cords.

Mainstem bronchi — The two air passageways connecting the trachea with the lungs.

Trachea — The "wind pipe" or air passageway extending from the throat to the mainstem bronchi.

Vallecula — A pouch formed by the base of the tongue and the epiglottis.

Vocal cords — Folds of mucous membrane on both sides of the trachea, just within the glottis.

When using the laryngoscope during intubation, the structures you actually see are shown here in an internal view of the oral cavity.

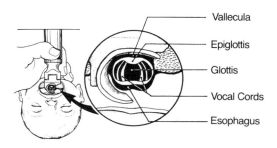

Positioning the Infant

Once the equipment is prepared, you are ready to intubate the infant. The first step is to position the infant for insertion of the laryngoscope blade.

The correct position of the infant for intubation is on a *flat* surface with the head in a midline position and the neck slightly extended. It may be helpful to place a roll under the baby's shoulders to maintain slight extension of the neck.

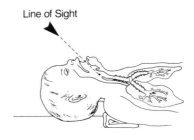

Infant in Correct Position

This position aligns the trachea for optimal viewing by allowing a straight line of sight into the glottis once the laryngoscope has been properly placed.

It is important not to hyperextend the neck as this will raise the trachea above your line of sight as well as narrow the trachea, thus limiting air entry.

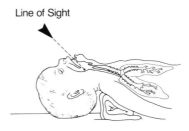

Neck Hyperextended

If the neck is not extended enough and the head is flexed toward the chest, you will not be able to directly visualize the trachea. This position also compromises air entry.

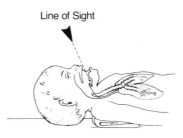

Neck Underextended

Correct and incorrect positions for endotracheal intubation are shown here.

Correct

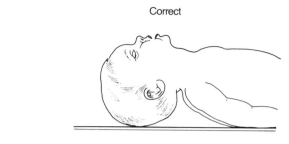

Neck Slightly Extended

Incorrect

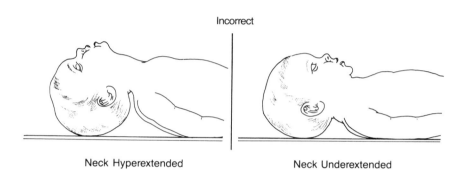

Neck Hyperextended   Neck Underextended

Practice Activity 2

This practice activity covers the anatomical landmarks and positioning of the infant.

Fill In

1–8. On the illustrations below you will see lines drawn to eight anatomical landmarks. Write the name of each in the corresponding space below.

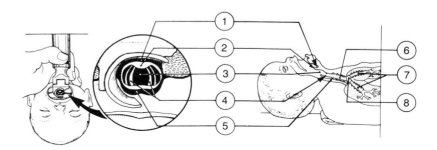

1. _____   5. _____

2. _____   6. _____

3. _____   7. _____

4. _____   8. _____

Select

9. Select the illustration below that shows the correct position of the infant for introduction of the laryngoscope and ET tube. _____

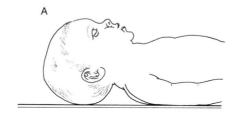

A

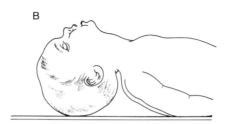

B

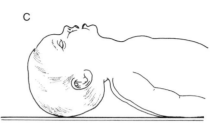

C

True/False

10. _____ The glottis is more easily visualized if the neck is hyperextended.

11. _____ During intubation, the infant should be on a flat surface.

Practice Activity 2: Answers

Compare your answers with those given here.

Fill In

1. Vallecula

2. Epiglottis

3. Glottis

4. Vocal Cords

5. Esophagus

6. Trachea

7. Mainstem bronchi

8. Carina

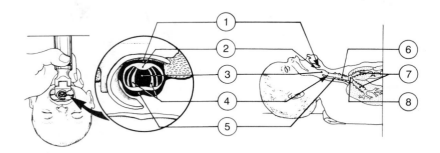

Select

9. C

True/False

10. **False**—In the neonate, hyperextension of the neck elevates the trachea above your line of sight.

11. **True**

Decision

If . . .	Then . . .
You were correct on all 11 items . . .	Excellent. You are ready to learn the specifics of the intubation procedure.
You missed any item . . .	Review carefully before continuing. Knowing the anatomy and proper positioning are essential to the intubation procedure.

Inserting the Laryngoscope and Visualizing the Glottis

As soon as the infant is properly positioned, the laryngoscope should be inserted, and the glottis (the opening to the trachea) visualized. This is the most difficult and critical part of the procedure. Once there is a clear view of the glottis, inserting an ET tube is accomplished relatively easily.

The steps used by the person intubating are given in detail here and in the following section for benefit of both the operator and assistant. Common knowledge of the procedure on the part of the operator and assistant facilitates the team work necessary to perform intubation quickly and efficiently.

Preparing for Insertion

Stand at the head of the infant. Turn on the laryngoscope light and hold the laryngoscope in your left hand between your thumb and the first three fingers with the blade pointing *away* from you.

Note:

The laryngoscope is designed to be held in the *left* hand—by both right- and left-handed individuals. If held in the right hand, the closed, curved part of the blade may block your view of the glottis, as well as make insertion of the ET tube impossible.

Stabilize the infant's head with your right hand.

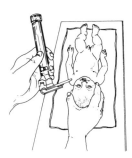

Introducing Blade

The goal in inserting the laryngoscope blade is to slide it over the tongue with the tip of the blade resting in the vallecula (the area between the base of the tongue and the epiglottis).

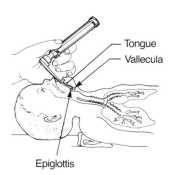

Tongue
Vallecula
Epiglottis

Exception:

In general, the blade should be placed in the vallecula. However, in extremely premature infants the vallecula may be too small, in which case it may be necessary to use the blade to *gently* lift the epiglottis.

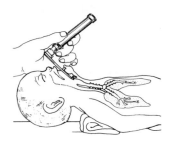

To properly position the blade, introduce the blade into the infant's mouth between the tongue and palate. Gently advance the tip to just beyond the base of the tongue.

Visualizing Glottis
Lift Blade

Once the blade is inserted the desired distance, lift it slightly, thus lifting the tongue out of the way to expose the pharyngeal area.

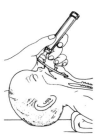 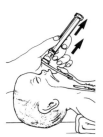

When lifting the blade, raise the *entire* blade by pulling up in the direction the handle is pointing. *Do not just lift the tip of the blade* by using a rocking motion and pulling the handle toward you. The latter will not produce the view of the glottis you desire and will put excessive pressure on the alveolar ridge and possibly harm future tooth formation.

Correct   Incorrect

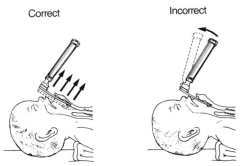

Assess Landmarks

With the blade properly inserted and slightly elevated, the pharyngeal area is exposed. The next step is to look for landmarks. It is important to identify *where* the tip of the blade is. This will enable you to take immediate corrective action (if necessary) in an attempt to visualize the glottis.

Correct Blade Position

If the tip is correctly positioned in the vallecula, you should see the epiglottis at the top with the glottic opening below.

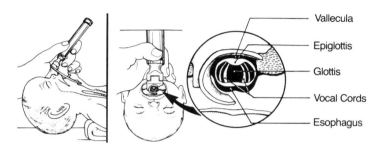

Vallecula
Epiglottis
Glottis
Vocal Cords
Esophagus

Properly Positioned in Vallecula

Incorrect Blade Position

An incorrectly positioned blade is either inserted too far, not far enough, or too far to the right or left. The landmarks that signal each of these positions are given here, along with the appropriate corrective action.

Position	Landmarks	Corrective Action
Not inserted far enough	You see the tongue surrounding the blade	Advance the blade farther

Position	**Landmarks**	**Corrective Action**
Inserted too far	You see the wall of the esophagus surrounding the blade	Withdraw the blade slowly until the epiglottis and glottis come into view

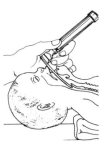 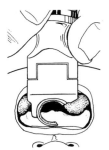 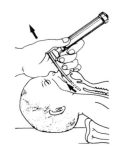

Position	**Landmarks**	**Corrective Action**
Inserted off to the side	In the posterior pharynx, you see part of the trachea to the side of the blade	Gently move the blade back to the midline, then advance or retreat according to the landmarks seen

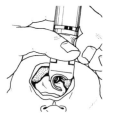 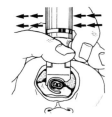

If these corrective measures fail to bring the epiglottis and glottis into view, withdraw the laryngoscope, ventilate the infant with a bag and mask, and begin again.

"STOP" After 20 Seconds!

To minimize hypoxia, intubation attempts should be limited to 20 seconds. The infant should be stabilized between attempts by ventilating with a bag and mask.

External Laryngeal Pressure

In some infants, particularly very small ones, pressure on the neck over the larynx will maximize the view of the glottis.

Before   After

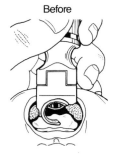 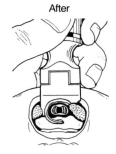

This is accomplished by using the fourth or fifth finger of the left hand, or asking an assistant to apply the pressure.

Applied by Assistant   Applied by Operator

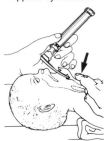 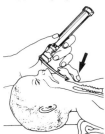

Suction PRN

When inserting the laryngoscope blade, if you encounter secretions blocking the airway, suction the area. Suctioning secretions is essential for visualizing the glottis and preventing aspiration, should the infant gasp.

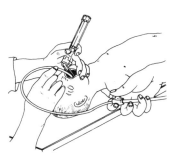

Summary

As stated earlier, the most difficult part of the procedure is obtaining an unobstructed view of the glottis. This involves the following steps:

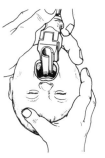

1. Insert blade to just beyond base of tongue.

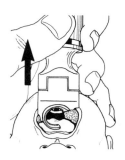

2. Lift the blade and identify landmarks.

Ideally, as you lift the blade, the glottis and epiglottis will come into view.

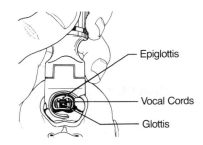

— Epiglottis

— Vocal Cords

— Glottis

---

3. If landmarks are not seen:
  • Determine blade placement:
    • On tongue?
    • In esophagus?
    • To the side?
  • Take corrective action, and reassess landmarks.
  • Use external laryngeal pressure if necessary to lower the trachea.
  • Use suction p.r.n. to clear airway.
  If 20 seconds have passed, stop and ventilate with a bag and mask.

Start

Stop

20 Seconds

Placing the Endotracheal Tube

Once the vocal cords and trachea are visualized, insert the endotracheal tube.

Inserting Tube

When you are able to visualize the glottis and vocal cords, follow these steps for inserting the endotracheal tube:

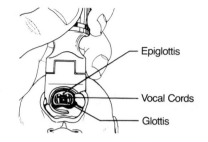

— Epiglottis

— Vocal Cords

— Glottis

1. Holding the tube in your right hand, introduce it into the right side of the infant's mouth. This will prevent the tube from blocking your view of the glottis.

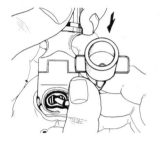

2. Keep the glottis in view, and when the vocal cords are apart, insert the tip of the ET tube until the vocal cord guide is at the level of the cords.

Insertion of ET Tube Between Cords

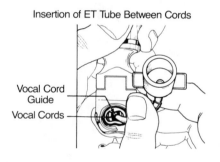

Vocal Cord Guide

Vocal Cords

This will position the tube in the trachea—approximately half way between the vocal cords and carina.

(If the cords are together, wait for them to open. Do not touch the closed cords with the tip of the tube as it may cause spasm of the cords. If the cords do not open before the 20-second limit has expired, stop and ventilate with a bag and mask.)

Vocal Cords — — Carina

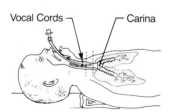

Note:

Some prefer using the "tip-to-lip" measurement for inserting the endotracheal tube the appropriate distance. A quick determination of the tip-to-lip distance can be obtained by adding "6" to the infant's weight in kg. The following chart is based on the infant's weight and can be used as a guide as to how far a tube should be inserted.

Weight	Depth of Insertion (cm from upper lip)
1 kg	7 cm
2 kg	8 cm
3 kg	9 cm
4 kg	10 cm

Removing Laryngoscope

3. With the right hand held against the face, hold the tube *firmly* at the lips. Use your left hand to *carefully* remove the laryngoscope without displacing the tube. If a stylet was used, then remove it from the endotracheal tube.

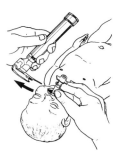

Checking Placement of Tube

4. The tube should be checked immediately to be sure it is properly positioned in the trachea. How this should be done will be discussed in the next section.

Practice Activity 3

The following questions cover the intubation procedure.

Fill In

Below are four views you may see after inserting and lifting the laryngoscope blade. For each, identify *where* the blade is positioned and describe the *corrective action* required, if one is necessary.

1. _____
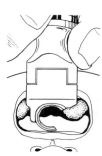
   (blade position)

2. _____
   (corrective action)

3. _____
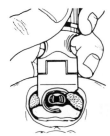
   (blade position)

4. _____
   (corrective action)

5. _____
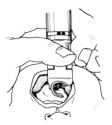
   (blade position)

6. _____
   (corrective action)

7. _____
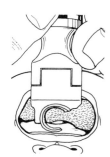
   (blade position)

8. _____
   (corrective action)

9. Pressure applied over the trachea during intubation tends to:

_____

_____

10. Each intubation attempt should be limited to _____ seconds.

Sequencing

11. Below is a list of steps for inserting the laryngoscope and ET tube during endotracheal intubation. Number the steps in the correct order (1 for the first step, 2 for the second, etc.).

_____ Insert the ET tube into the glottis.

_____ Stabilize the infant's head.

_____ Insert the blade between the tongue and palate to just beyond the base of the tongue.

_____ Pick up the laryngoscope and turn on the light.

_____ Lift the blade and visualize the epiglottis and glottis.

True/False

12. _____ The laryngoscope is always held in the left hand regardless of whether the person is right- or left-handed.

13. _____ In general, when intubating neonates, the tip of the laryngoscope should be inserted in the vallecula, rather than used to lift the epiglottis.

14. _____ If the tip of the laryngoscope is positioned in the vallecula, you should not expect to see the epiglottis.

15. _____ When you lift the laryngoscope blade to improve your view of the glottis, you should pull the laryngoscope handle toward you.

16. _____ If after inserting and lifting the laryngoscope you do not *immediately* see the glottis, you should remove the laryngoscope and try again.

17. _____ When inserting the ET tube, care should be taken to prevent blocking your view of the glottis.

Practice Activity 3: Answers

Compare your answers with those given below.

Fill In

1. In too far

2. Retreat or withdraw the blade

3. Correct position

4. None

5. Off to the side

6. Move the blade back to midline position

7. Not in far enough

8. Advance the blade

9. Laryngeal pressure tends to lower the glottis, bringing it into view

10. 20 seconds

Sequencing

11. 5

    2

    3

    1

    4

True/False

12. **True**

13. **True**

14. **False** — You will see the epiglottis just below the tip of the blade.

15. **False** — You should lift the blade by pulling up on the laryngoscope handle, in the direction the handle is pointing.

16. **False** — You should quickly identify anatomical landmarks and take the appropriate corrective action. Pressure over the trachea may also help bring the glottis into view. If you still do not see the glottis *or* time to attempt intubation has exceeded 20 seconds, you will need to withdraw the blade and ventilate the infant before trying again.

17. **True**

Decision

If . . .	Then . . .
You answered all the items correctly, or missed no more than 1 . . .	Good! You are ready to continue.
You missed 2 or more questions . . .	Stop and carefully review the appropriate information. This practice activity covers material essential to the intubation procedure.

Confirming ET Tube Placement

If the ET tube has been inserted for positive-pressure ventilation (vs. tracheal suctioning), the position of the tube must be confirmed. Initially, you should listen for bilateral breath sounds and observe for bilateral chest movement. Later, when the situation permits, confirmation of the tube's position may be made by obtaining a chest x-ray.

Initial Confirmation

Listen for Breath Sounds

Immediately after removing the laryngoscope blade, while holding the tube firmly in place, you must check the location of the tip of the tube. This is accomplished by attaching a resuscitation bag to the ET tube connector and ventilating the infant. This requires two people—one to ventilate the infant and the other to listen to both sides of the chest and over the stomach with a stethoscope. If the tube is correctly placed, you will hear:

- Air entering *both* sides of the chest and
- Breath sounds of equal intensity.

No air will be heard entering the stomach.

Note:

When listening to breath sounds, be sure to place your stethoscope laterally and high on the chest wall. If the stethoscope is placed lower, you are more likely to mistake air entering the stomach for breath sounds.

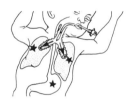

Three Areas to Listen for Air Entry
(Air should be entering both lungs, not stomach)

Observe Abdomen and Chest

In addition to listening for breath sounds, observe the chest and abdomen. If the tube is positioned correctly, you will see:

- A rise of the *chest,* and
- *No* gastric distention with ventilation.

Correct Placement

If the tube is correctly placed in the mid-tracheal region, there should be:

Signs

- Bilateral breath sounds
- Equal breath sounds
- Slight rise of the chest with each ventilation
- *No* air heard entering stomach
- *No* gastric distention

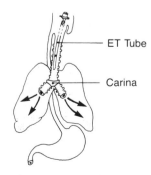

Correctly Placed Tube

Two Actions

1. *Note the cm mark on the tube at the level of the upper lip.* This will help you recognize if the tube moves.

2. *Secure the tube to the infant's face.* There are several ways this can be done, using either adhesive tape or an adhesive-backed endotracheal tube holder. In either event, the face should be dried thoroughly. Tincture of benzoin may be used to ensure adherence of the tape and to protect the skin. Ask someone to show you the technique used in your hospital for initially securing the tube. A more permanent fastening can be done later if an x-ray confirms correct placement and if long-term ventilation is required.

Incorrect Placement

If the tube is incorrectly placed, it is either in a mainstem bronchus or in the esophagus. Signs you would expect and the action that you should take are given for each situation.

Tube in Mainstem Bronchus

Signs

- Unilateral breath sounds
- Unequal breath sounds
- *No* air heard entering stomach
- *No* gastric distention

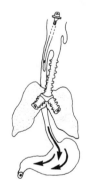

Action

Withdraw the tube approximately 1 cm and recheck placement.

Tube in Esophagus

Signs

- No breath sounds heard
- Air heard entering stomach
- Gastric distention may be seen

Action

Remove the tube, oxygenate the infant with a bag and mask, and reintroduce the ET tube.

Final Confirmation

If the ET tube is to remain in the trachea beyond the initial resuscitation, a chest film must be obtained for confirmation of correct tube position.

Correctly Positioned

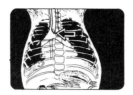

ET Tube in the Trachea, Above the Carina

Incorrectly Positioned

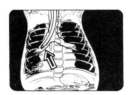   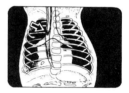

Tube in Right Mainstem Bronchus   Tube in Esophagus

Additional Step
Shorten Tube

After confirmation of correct tube position, if the ET tube extends *more than 4 cm* from the infant's lips, the tube should be shortened and the connector replaced. This will probably be necessary only in very small infants. Shortening the tube reduces the amount of dead space and lessens the chance of the tube becoming kinked.

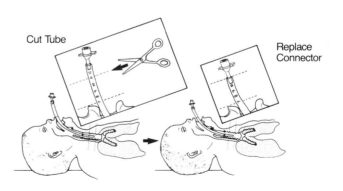

Cut Tube   Replace Connector

Practice Activity 4

The following practice activity will test your knowledge of the steps taken once the ET tube has been inserted.

Fill In

1. Where should the tip of the ET tube lie within the trachea?

_____

State the steps that should be taken to confirm correct placement.

2–3. *Initial Confirmation*

• _____

_____

• _____

_____

4. *Final Confirmation*

• _____

5. Draw an "X" on each of the three places you would place your stethoscope to listen for air entry when checking for correct ET tube placement.

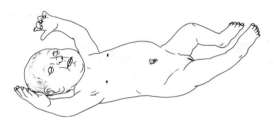

For each of the following descriptions, draw in *where* the ET tube is most likely positioned.

6. Breath sounds cannot be heard on either side of the chest. You think you hear air entering the stomach. There is abdominal movement each time the infant is ventilated.

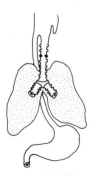

7. Breath sounds can be heard on both sides of the chest, but they sound much louder on the right side. No air is heard entering the stomach. You look closely for chest or abdominal movement, but cannot be sure of seeing any.

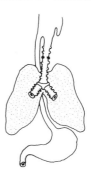

8. This time there is a slight rise and fall of the chest. No air can be heard entering the stomach. You hear breath sounds on both sides of the chest and they are equal in intensity.

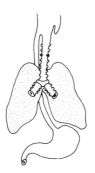

List in proper order the two steps that should be taken as soon as initial confirmation of correct tube placement has been obtained.

9. _____

10. _____

11. What additional step may need to be taken following confirmation of correct tube position?

_____

Practice Activity 4: Answers

Compare your answers with those given below.

Fill In

1. When correctly placed, the tip of the ET tube should lie within the *middle third* of the trachea (or half way between the vocal cords and the carina).

2–3. Initial Confirmation

- Use a stethoscope to listen to both sides of the chest and over the abdomen.

- Observe the chest and abdomen for movement

4. Final Confirmation

- Obtain a chest x-ray

5.

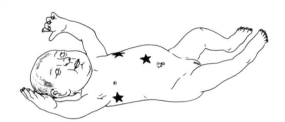

6.

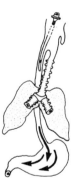

(Tube in Esophagus)

7.

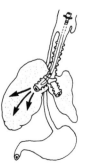

(Tube in Right Mainstem Bronchus)

8.

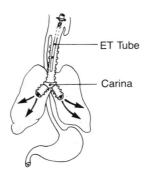

ET Tube

Carina

(Tube Properly Positioned in Trachea)

9. Note the cm mark on the tube at the level of the upper lip.

10. Tape tube to the infant's face.

11. Shortening tube so that no more than 4 cm extends beyond infant's lips.

Decision

If . . .	Then . . .
You answered them all correctly . . .	Good!
You missed any . . .	Carefully review the section on "Confirming ET Tube Placement."

Complications of the Procedure

A number of complications can result from endotracheal intubation in neonates. Intubation can produce or increase hypoxia, cause trauma to tissues, and introduce infection. However, when one is skilled in the procedure, the incidence of complications is minimized.

Study the following list: note some of the common causes of the complications.

Complication	Causes
Hypoxia	Taking too long to intubate
	Incorrect placement of tube
Bradycardia/Apnea	Hypoxia
	Vagal response due to the laryngoscope blade, ET tube, or suction catheter stimulating the posterior pharynx
Pneumothorax	Overventilation of one lung due to placement of tube in a main bronchus (usually the right)
Contusions or lacerations of tongue, gums, pharynx, epiglottis, trachea, vocal cords, or esophagus	Rough handling of laryngoscope or ET tube
	Laryngoscope blade that is too long or too short
Perforation of trachea or esophagus	Insertion of tube or stylet is too vigorous, or stylet protrudes beyond end of tube
Infection	Introduction of organisms via equipment or hands

Minimizing Hypoxia During Intubation

During intubation it is important not to induce or increase hypoxia. Thus it is important to know the steps that should be taken to prevent or minimize hypoxia *during* the procedure. These include:

• Providing free-flow oxygen, and

• Limiting intubation attempts to 20 seconds.

Using Free-Flow Oxygen

If an infant is making a respiratory effort, free-flow oxygen should be provided. A tube with oxygen flowing at 5 liters per minute should be held by the assistant as close to the infant's mouth and nose as possible without interfering with the procedure. Flow rates greater than 5 liters per minute are not necessary and will cool the infant if the oxygen has not been heated.

Limit to 20 Seconds

If intubation has not been successfully accomplished within 20 seconds of initially inserting the laryngoscope blade, the procedure should be stopped and the infant stabilized by ventilating with a bag and mask.

Start

Stop

20 Seconds

Role of the Assistant

An assistant, knowledgeable in the procedure and experienced in assisting with a number of intubations, is invaluable to the operator.

So far you have learned all that is expected of the assistant. Here is a summary of the assistant's role.

Before Intubation

Prepare and check equipment:
- ET Tube
- Laryngoscope
- Bag and Mask
- Oxygen Equipment
- Suction Equipment
- Tape or ET Tube Holder

During Intubation

Stabilize head, restraining infant if necessary

Hand equipment to operator: laryngoscope, ET tube, suction catheter, etc.

Provide free-flow oxygen *if* the infant is making a respiratory effort

Assist with suction catheter
- Select appropriate size catheter
- Occlude finger hole, on request

Provide pressure over trachea, on request

Monitor infant's heart rate, respiratory effort, and color

Monitor time spent in intubation attempt

Notify operator of intubation attempts exceeding 20 seconds

Assist with bag-and-mask ventilation if needed to stabilize infant between intubation attempts

Following Intubation

Hold tube securely to prevent displacement, if requested

Check tube placement
- Attach resuscitation bag to tube
- Ventilate, if requested
- Listen with stethoscope to both sides of chest and over stomach while infant is being ventilated
- Observe chest and abdomen for movement

Note cm marking on the tube at level of upper lip

Tape tube to face

Shorten tube if more than 4 cm extends from lips

Assist with positive-pressure ventilation

Plan Ahead

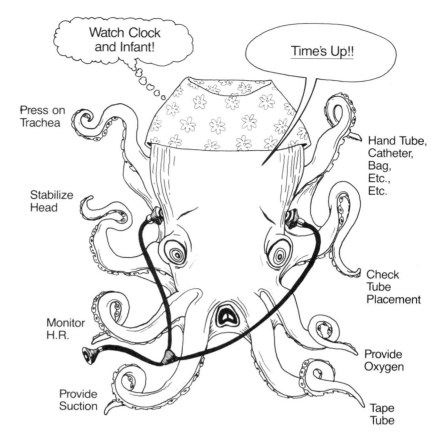

As an assistant, you may sometimes wish that, like an octopus, you had eight arms. But in reality, everything does not need to be done at the same time, nor is everything required for each infant. If time has been taken to properly prepare for the procedure, everything will be close at hand and often you will find that you will be able to concentrate on one activity at a time. With practice, you will be able to provide what is required and at the same time monitor the infant's condition.

Practice

If you will be assuming the role of assistant, use the checklist on page 5-67 to practice. You will be taken through the checklist by your instructor once you have completed the posttest.

Practice Activity 5

This is the final practice activity. Do your best in answering the following questions.

Completion

1–4. List four complications that can result from endotracheal intubation.

* _____

* _____

* _____

* _____

5–6. What two actions should be taken to prevent or minimize hypoxia *during* intubation?

* _____

_____

* _____

_____

True/False

7. _____ An experienced assistant does not need to prepare supplies/ equipment ahead of time to assist with endotracheal intubation.

8. _____ The chances of complications occurring with intubation are significantly reduced if both the operator and assistant perform their respective roles in a knowledgeable and skillful manner.

9. _____ The performance of a truly skilled operator is not enhanced by a skilled assistant.

10. _____ Endotracheal intubation must be practiced regularly if one is to maintain skill in performing the procedure.

Practice Activity 5: Answers

Compare your answers with those given below.

Completion

1–4. (Any four of the following)
Hypoxia
Bradycardia
Apnea
Vagal response
Contusions/lacerations of tongue, gums, pharynx, epiglottis, trachea, vocal cords, or esophagus
Perforation of esophagus or trachea
Infection
Pneumothorax

5–6. • Provide free-flow oxygen
• Limit intubation attempts to 20 seconds

True/False

7. **False** — If supplies and equipment have not been prepared ahead of time, precious time is lost in doing so during the procedure.

8. **True**

9. **False** — The performance of even a truly skilled operator can be enhanced by a skilled assistant.

10. **True**

Decision

If ...	Then ...
You answered all items correctly ...	Go on to the review and posttest.
You missed any ...	Be sure you understand the correct answers before continuing.

Review

Before you proceed to the posttest, review the steps involved in intubating a neonate.

Obtain and Prepare Supplies and Equipment

Obtain the supplies and equipment and prepare them in the following way:

Select the appropriate ET tube size based on the infant's weight or gestational age.

Weight	Gestational Age	Size
Below 1000 gm	Below 28 weeks	2.5 mm
1000–2000 gm	28–34 weeks	3.0 mm
2000–3000 gm	34–38 weeks	3.5 mm
Above 3000 gm	Above 38 weeks	3.5–4.0 mm

ET Tube

To prepare the ET tube:
- Cut the tube at the 13-cm mark.
- Replace the ET tube connector.
- Insert stylet the appropriate distance and secure its position (optional).

Laryngoscope

To prepare the laryngoscope:
- Select the correct size blade (No. 0 for preterm, No. 1 for fullterm) and attach it to laryngoscope.
- Check the light, and replace batteries or bulb if required.

Additional Items

To complete the preparations:
- Cut strip(s) of tape or obtain ET tube holder.
- Prepare suction equipment:

  Maximum suction pressures
  100 mm Hg
  or
  4 in Hg.
- Prepare tubing with 100% oxygen.
- Prepare resuscitation bag and mask.

Position Infant

Position infant flat with the neck slightly extended.

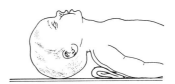

Insert Laryngoscope

Stand at the head of the infant. Be sure the laryngoscope blade is locked in operating position, and hold the laryngoscope in the left hand. Stabilize the infant's head with the right hand.

Introduce the blade into the mouth and advance it to just beyond the base of the tongue. This should position the blade in the vallecula.

Visualize Glottis

Lift the blade and observe for landmarks. As you lift the blade, the epiglottis and the glottis should come into view.

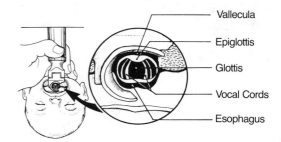

- Vallecula
- Epiglottis
- Glottis
- Vocal Cords
- Esophagus

If the glottis and epiglottis do not come into view, additional steps must be taken. You will need to ask one or more of the following questions and then take the appropriate action.

- **What landmarks do you see?** If blade is in too far, not far enough, or off to the side, take corrective action.

- **Is view of glottis obscured by secretions?** Suction secretions.

- **Do you feel blade is properly positioned, but you do not see glottic opening, or you see only posterior portion?** Apply tracheal pressure to lower the trachea.

Inserting ET Tube

When the glottis can be seen, introduce the ET tube into the right side of the mouth and into the glottic opening.

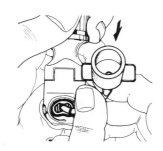

Insert the tip of the tube until the vocal cord guide is at the level of the vocal cords.

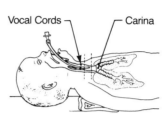

Check Placement

When the tube is positioned, hold the tube in place as you carefully withdraw the laryngoscope and stylet.

Initial Confirmation

Next, attach a resuscitation bag to the tube's connector and ventilate the infant. A second person is needed to listen with a stethoscope to both sides of the chest and over the stomach.

- **Bilateral breath sounds** of equal intensity, with no air heard entering the stomach, indicate that the tube's tip is correctly positioned. Note cm marking at level of upper lip. Then stabilize the tube by taping it to the infant's face.

- **Unilateral or unequal breath sounds** indicate that the tube's tip is located in one of the mainstem bronchi. **Withdraw the tube approximately 1 cm** and check the breath sounds again. If in a mainstem bronchus, no air will be heard entering stomach.

- If **no breath sounds** can be detected in the lungs and air can be heard entering stomach, the tube has probably been placed in the esophagus. **Withdraw** the tube and reinsert it after oxygenating the infant with bag and mask.

- **Observe the chest and abdomen.** If tube is properly positioned, with ventilation you should see a slight rise of the chest and no gastric distention.

Follow-Up Confirmation

After initial confirmation of correct placement, the tube is affixed to the infant's face, and a chest x-ray must be obtained for final confirmation of tube placement.

Overview of the Procedure

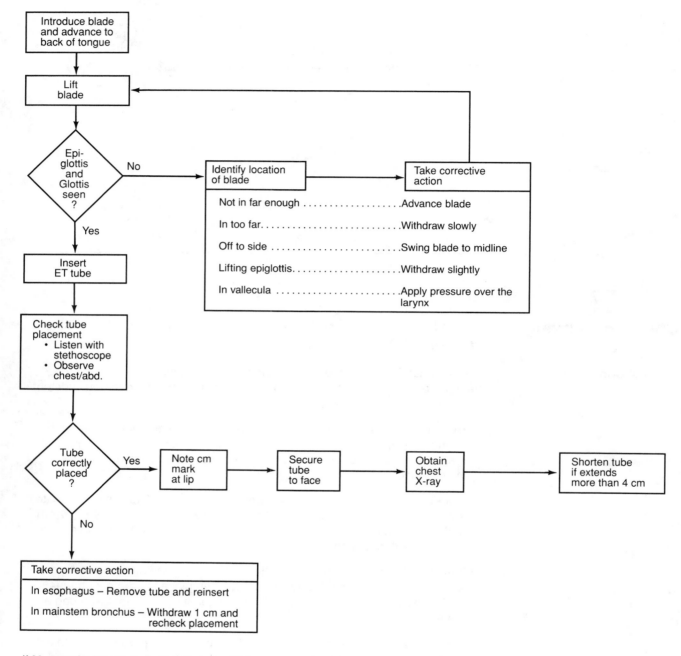

```
Introduce blade
and advance to
back of tongue
        │
        ▼
     Lift
     blade  ◄─────────────────────────────────────────┐
        │                                              │
        ▼                                              │
   Epi-                                                │
   glottis         No      Identify location    Take corrective
   and      ──────────►    of blade        ───► action
   Glottis
   seen                    Not in far enough ................Advance blade
   ?
   │ Yes                   In too far........................Withdraw slowly
   ▼
   Insert                  Off to side ......................Swing blade to midline
   ET tube
   │                       Lifting epiglottis................Withdraw slightly
   ▼
   Check tube              In vallecula .....................Apply pressure over the
   placement                                                 larynx
   • Listen with
     stethoscope
   • Observe
     chest/abd.
        │
        ▼
   Tube          Yes    Note cm       Secure      Obtain      Shorten tube
   correctly  ──────►   mark    ───►  tube   ───► chest  ───► if extends
   placed               at lip        to face     X-ray       more than 4 cm
   ?
   │ No
   ▼
Take corrective action

In esophagus – Remove tube and reinsert

In mainstem bronchus – Withdraw 1 cm and
                       recheck placement
```

If 20 seconds since blade first introduced and tube not properly positioned
- Remove laryngoscope, and
- Ventilate with bag and mask using 100% oxygen

Posttest
Lesson 5 — Endotracheal Intubation

Name _____ Date _____

This posttest is for both the assistant and the person performing intubation. Before you go on to the practice portion of this lesson, test yourself on the key concepts regarding endotracheal intubation. Follow the directions for each section.

Selection

1–4. From the following situations, select those in which endotracheal intubation is definitely indicated. _____

A. Infants with a 1-minute Apgar score of 3 or below

B. Infants in whom bag and mask fails to provide adequate ventilation

C. Infants with thick meconium in the amniotic fluid

D. All apneic, premature infants less than 32 weeks

E. Infants suspected of having a diaphragmatic hernia

F. Infants requiring prolonged positive-pressure ventilation

Completion

Indicate the correct ET tube size for infants with the following weights:

Weight		Tube Size
5. 800 gm	—	_____ mm
6. 3400 gm	—	_____ mm
7. 1200 gm	—	_____ mm
8. 2500 gm	—	_____ mm
9. 4200 gm	—	_____ mm
10. 1800 gm	—	_____ mm

State the three steps involved in preparing an endotracheal tube for insertion, once a tube of the correct size has been selected.

11. _____

12. _____

13. _____

14–15. State the two steps involved in preparing a laryngoscope for use.

• _____

• _____

16–19. List the four additional items needed to assure that adequate equipment and supplies are available when intubating a neonate.

- _____

- _____

- _____

- _____

20. State the suction pressure that should not be exceeded in suctioning secretions during intubation. State the pressure in terms that relate to how your gauge measures pressure. Include the correct unit of measurement (mm Hg or in Hg). _____

Selection

21. Select the illustration below that shows the correct position of the infant for introduction of the laryngoscope and ET tube. _____

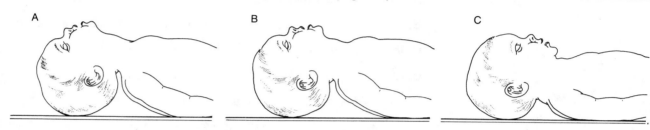

A   B   C

Sequencing

22. Below is a list of steps for inserting the laryngoscope and ET tube during endotracheal intubation. Number the steps in the correct order (1 for the first step, 2 for the second, etc.).

_____ Insert the ET tube into the glottis.

_____ Stabilize the infant's head.

_____ Insert the blade between the tongue and palate to just beyond the base of the tongue.

_____ Pick up the laryngoscope and turn on the light.

_____ Lift the blade and visualize the epiglottis and glottis.

Selection

23. Select the illustration that demonstrates the correct way to *lift* the laryngoscope blade in order to improve your view of the glottis. _____

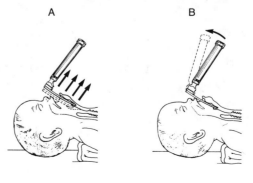

A   B

Fill In

24–31. On the illustrations below, you will see lines drawn to eight anatomical landmarks. Write the name of each in the corresponding space below.

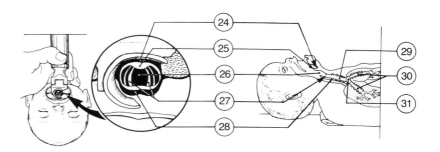

24. _____   28. _____

25. _____   29. _____

26. _____   30. _____

27. _____   31. _____

Identify

Study the four internal views below and identify *where* the blade is positioned and the corrective action required, if one is necessary. Write the letter(s) of your selection in the spaces provided.

Blade Positions

A. To the side
B. Correct position
C. Not in far enough
D. In too far

Corrective Actions

E. Advance blade
F. Withdraw blade
G. Move blade to midline position

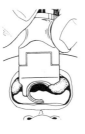 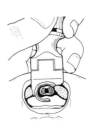 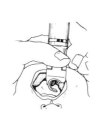 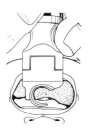

32. _____   33. _____   34. _____   35. _____

Fill In

36–37. What two actions should be taken to prevent or minimize hypoxia *during* intubation?

- _____

  _____

- _____

  _____

State the steps that should be taken to confirm correct endotracheal tube placement.

38–39. Initial Confirmation

- _____

  _____

- _____

  _____

40. Final Confirmation

- _____

41. Draw an "X" on each of the three places you would place your stethoscope to listen for air entry when checking for correct ET tube placement.

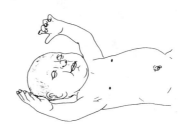

For each of the following descriptions state *where* the ET tube is most likely positioned.

42. Breath sounds can be heard on both sides of the chest, but they sound much louder on the right. You do not see any chest or abdominal movement.

_____

43. You hear breath sounds on both sides of the chest that are equal in intensity. You do not hear air entering the stomach. There is a rise of the chest with each ventilation.

_____

44. Breath sounds cannot be heard on either side of the chest. You hear air entering the stomach. Each time the infant is ventilated, there is abdominal movement.

_____

List, in proper order, the two steps that should be taken as soon as initial confirmation of correct tube placement has been obtained.

45. _____

46. _____

47. What additional step may need to be taken following final confirmation of correct tube placement?

_____

48–51. List four complications that can result from endotracheal intubation.

- _____

- _____

- _____

- _____

Lesson 5 Posttest: Answers

Compare your answers with those given below.

Selection

1–4. **B, C, E, F**

Completion

   5. 800 gm — 2.5 mm

   6. 3400 gm — 3.5–4.0 mm

   7. 1200 gm — 3.0 mm

   8. 2500 gm — 3.5 mm

   9. 4200 gm — 3.5–4.0 mm

 10. 1800 gm — 3.0 mm

 11. Shorten tube to 13 cm

 12. Replace ET tube connector

 13. Insert stylet (optional)

14–15. • Attach correct size blade
        • Check light

16–19. • Adhesive tape
        • Suction equipment
        • Oxygen equipment
        • Resuscitation bag and mask

 20. 100 mm Hg or 4 in Hg

Selection

21. B

Sequencing

22. 5
    2
    3
    1
    4

Selection

23. A

Fill In

24. Vallecula   **28.** Esophagus
25. Epiglottis   **29.** Trachea
26. Glottis   **30.** Mainstem bronchi
27. Vocal cords   **31.** Carina

Identify

32. D, F   **33. B**   **34. A, G**   **35. C, E**

Fill In

36–37. • Provide free-flow oxygen
• Limit intubation attempts to 20 seconds

38–39. Initial Confirmation
• Use a stethoscope to listen to both sides of chest and over the abdomen
• Observe the chest and abdomen for movement

40. Final Confirmation
• Obtain a chest x-ray

41.

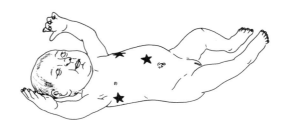

42. In right mainstem bronchus

43. In trachea

44. In esophagus

45. Note the cm mark on the tube at the level of the upper lip

46. Tape tube to the infant's face

47. Shorten tube so that no more than 4 cm extends beyond infant's lips

48–51. (Any four of the following)

• Hypoxia
• Bradycardia
• Apnea
• Vagal response
• Contusions/lacerations
• Perforation of esophagus or trachea
• Infection
• Pneumothorax

Decision

If . . .	Then . . .
You had at least 46 correct answers . . .	You have successfully completed the posttest. If you will be assisting, go on to the "Performance Checklist" for assistants on page 5-67. If you will actually perform intubations, go on to the "Practice Guide for Intubation" on the next page.
You missed more than 5 questions . . .	Review any information related to the items you missed. If you have any questions, see your instructor or supervisor. When you have mastered the material, take the posttest again.

Practice Guide for Intubation

Now that you have passed the posttest on the intubation procedure, it's time to proceed to the manual skills involved. Learning to manipulate the equipment, visualize the landmarks, and insert the endotracheal tube can be accomplished using either of the following:

- An infant resuscitation manikin that permits insertion of an ET tube under direct vision, or
- An appropriately anesthetized animal model.

It is suggested that you first use the intubation manikin until you become adept in the steps.

Prepare Practice Area

Set up your practice area so that the manikin, equipment, and lesson are in front of you.

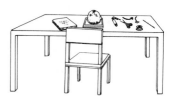

Equipment and Supplies

You will need the following equipment and supplies to practice the intubation procedure.

Intubation manikin

Or other simulation

Laryngoscope

With fresh batteries and functioning light source

Blade

No. 1 (fullterm) if using the intubation manikin

ET tube

(Actual size should be determined by the size of the manikin you are using)

Stylet

Oxygen tubing

Suction device

With 10–12 Fr. catheter

Adhesive tape

1/2" or 3/4" roll

Scissors

Resuscitation bag

For initial confirmation of tube placement

Stethoscope

To listen for breath sounds if using an anesthetized animal model

Clock

With a sweep second hand

Prepare Equipment

Prepare ET tube:
- Cut tube at 13 cm
- Replace connector
- Insert stylet (optional)
  - Tip should not protrude from ET tube
  - Should be secured so it cannot advance farther into tube

Prepare Laryngoscope:
- Attach blade to handle and check light source
  - Replace batteries or bulb if necessary

Prepare additional items:
- Cut strip(s) of adhesive tape
- Check resuscitation bag for function

Landmark Practice

Before proceeding, you should practice identifying, on the manikin, some of the anatomical landmarks discussed earlier in this lesson. The best way to do this is to purposefully place the blade in the manikin incorrectly so that you can see what it looks like when the laryngoscope blade is:

- Not in far enough
- In too far
- To one side
- Lifting the epiglottis, instead of resting in the vallecula

The following pages contain illustrations showing each of these four situations. Using the manikin, you should attempt to simulate each of the interior views shown.

Get Ready

Position properly—If using an intubation manikin or anesthetized animal, position flat on the back with neck slightly extended. Use a roll under the shoulders, if necessary, to maintain the head in the correct position.

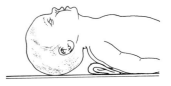

Hold laryngoscope—Using your left hand, hold the handle between your thumb and first three fingers. Point blade *away* from you.

Stand at the infant's head and stabilize the head with your right hand.

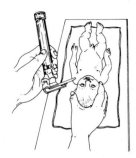

Now you are ready to insert the blade between the tongue and palate to obtain the following views.

Not in Far Enough

This is what you will see when the laryngoscope blade is *not inserted far enough.* The tip of the blade is positioned on the tongue. Note that you can see tongue beyond the tip of the blade. You may or may not be able to see the tip of the epiglottis below the tongue.

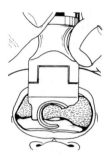

Corrective action: You probably recall that when the blade is not inserted far enough you should advance it farther toward the base of the tongue.

In Too Far

When the blade is *inserted too far* your view will be that of the esophagus. This is what it will look like. Note that in this view you do not see any of the structures that you would need to see for intubation—the epiglottis, glottis, or vocal cords. You may see some of the tongue to the side(s) of the laryngoscope.

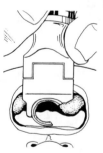

Corrective action: When this view is identified during the procedure, you should withdraw the blade slowly until the glottis and epiglottis come into view.

Off to One Side

Although the blade may be introduced at the midline position, the tip may be off to the side. You would therefore see only part of the desired structures (the epiglottis and glottis) or see them off to the side of the tip of the blade. Using the manikin, move the blade to the side to simulate this view. Also, move the blade to see what it would look like if positioned on the opposite side.

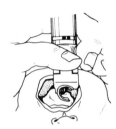

Corrective action: Gently maneuver the blade back to the midline position. Then advance or retreat according to the landmarks seen.

Lifting the Epiglottis

In general, the blade should be in the vallecula, although in very small infants it may be necessary to use the tip to lift the epiglottis. Attempt to simulate this view in the manikin. Note that the glottis can be seen, but not the epiglottis. You should be able to quickly detect if the blade is lifting the epiglottis rather than the vallecula.

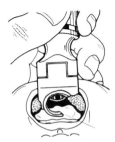

Corrective action: To position the tip in the vallecula, retreat *slowly* until the epiglottis can be seen.

Desired View

Here is a reminder of the visual landmarks you should expect to see when the laryngoscope blade is properly inserted in the vallecula and the blade has been lifted.

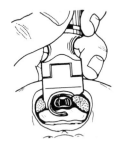

The Procedure

With the laryngoscope in the left hand and the right hand used to stabilize the head, go through the procedure as you would on a live infant. The practice you completed will help you detect correct and incorrect placement of the laryngoscope blade.

Insert Laryngoscope

1. Introduce the blade and advance it to the base of the tongue.

Lift Blade

2. Lift the laryngoscope blade. Are you lifting the blade correctly by pulling upward in the direction the handle is pointing rather than tilting the handle back toward you?

Assess Placement

3. Assess landmarks.

   What anatomical structures do you see?

   Where is the tip of the blade positioned?
   • On the tongue?
   • In too far?
   • To the side?
   • Lifting the epiglottis?
   • In the vallecula?

Corrective Action

4. Take corrective action, if necessary, and reassess blade location.

View Glottis

5. With blade properly inserted in the vallecula and lifted, obtain a clear view of the glottis and vocal cords.

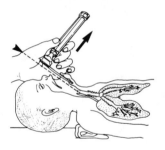

Laryngeal Pressure

In an infant, visualization of the glottis may require that pressure be applied over the larynx. This can be done by using the fifth finger of your left hand or by asking another person to apply pressure.

Practice applying laryngeal pressure, although doing so on the intubation head may not result in lowering the glottis since the positions of the structures are fixed.

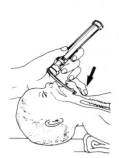

Insert ET Tube

6. When you are able to visualize the glottis and vocal cords, insert the ET tube, keeping the glottis in view.
   - Did you introduce the tube into right side of mouth?
   - Did you keep the vocal cord guide in view?
   - Did you stop inserting the ET tube when the vocal cord guide reached the level of the vocal cords?

Remove Laryngoscope

7. With the ET tube inserted, *carefully* remove the laryngoscope while holding the tube securely in place with your right hand.

Remove Stylet

If a stylet is used, remove it while continuing to hold the ET tube securely.

Confirm Tube Placement

8. How you initially confirm tube placement will depend on whether you are using an intubation manikin or appropriately anesthetized animal model.

Intubation Manikin

Most intubation manikins have balloons that represent the lungs. If the ET tube is placed in the trachea, both "lungs" will inflate when PPV is given via the resuscitation bag. If only one balloon inflates, or if neither inflates, immediate corrective action is indicated.

Anesthetized Animal Model

Using an appropriately anesthetized animal model allows you to confirm tube placement as you would in a live infant. Ventilate with the resuscitation bag and listen for air entry over both sides of the chest and over the stomach. Also observe for chest and abdominal movement.

Secure Tube

9. Complete the procedure by:
   - Noting the cm mark at the level of the upper lip.
   - Securing the tube to the face. If properly secured, a moderate "tug" on the tube should not cause displacement.

In intubating a live infant, what two additional steps would need to be taken?

You were correct if you thought of:

1. Obtaining an x-ray for final confirmation of placement, and

2. Checking to see if the tube needs shortening so that no more than 4 cm extends from the lips.

Continue Practice

Continue practicing intubation until you feel comfortable with the equipment and the procedure and you are able to correctly place the tube within the allotted 20 seconds.

Performance Checklist
Lesson 5—Assisting With Endotracheal Intubation

Instructions

Instructor: Using an infant resuscitation manikin (not an intubation head) have the participant demonstrate each of the steps on the checklist.

Judge the performance of each step carried out, and check (✔) when the action is completed correctly. If done incorrectly, circle the box so that you can discuss that step later.

Equipment and Supplies

Infant resuscitation manikin (not an intubation head)
Shoulder roll
Laryngoscope with fresh batteries and functioning bulb
Blade — No. 0 and 1
ET tubes — 2.5, 3.0, 3.5, 4.0 mm
Stylet
Adhesive tape — 1/2″ or 3/4″ roll
Scissors
Oxygen tubing
Suction device — suction setup with 10 Fr., or larger,
    suction catheter
Resuscitation bag and mask
Stethoscope

Performance Checklist
Lesson 5 — Assisting With Endotracheal Intubation

Name _____ Instructor _____ Date _____

You will be asked by your instructor to demonstrate each of the steps on this checklist.

Preparing for Intubation

Instructor: "Prepare the supplies and equipment needed for intubating an infant weighing _____ grams."

ET Tube

☐ **1. Selects correct size tube**

☐ **2. Cuts tube at 13 cm**

☐ **3. Replaces connector, securing a tight fit**

☐ **4. Inserts stylet**
- Stylet tip is well *within* tip of tube
- Secures stylet

Laryngoscope

☐ **5. Selects appropriate size blade**

☐ **6. Attaches blade to laryngoscope and checks light**

☐ **7. Takes appropriate action if light does not work**
- Changes batteries and/or bulb
- Obtains another laryngoscope

Additional Equipment

☐ **8. Cuts strip(s) of tape**

☐ **9. Obtains bag and mask**
- Bag checked for function
- Bag provides 90–100% O_2
- Selects appropriate size mask

☐ **10. Prepares tubing with 100% O_2**

☐ **11. Prepares suction equipment**

Assisting with Intubation

Instructor: Ask the student to demonstrate each of the following:

☐ **12. Positioning the infant**
- Infant flat
- Neck slightly extended

☐ **13. Providing free-flow oxygen**

☐ **14. Applying laryngeal pressure**

☐ **15. Confirming tube placement**
(Instructor will need to provide PPV)
- Places stethoscope over appropriate three areas
- States what one would expect to *hear* if the tube is correctly placed
- States that one would observe chest and abdomen for movement and what one would expect to *see* if tube is correctly placed

☐ **16. Securing tube to face**
- Holds tube in position while securing
- Reports cm marking at level of upper lip
- Maintains position of tube during securing of tube
- Uses correct procedure
- Tube maintains position when "tugged" by instructor
- Shortens tube if more than 4 cm extends from lips

Performance Checklist
Lesson 5 — Performing Endotracheal Intubation

Instructions

Instructor: To complete this checklist, the participant must go through the procedure twice, completing all steps satisfactorily. Because much of this procedure cannot be viewed directly by the instructor (from insertion of the laryngoscope through placement of the ET tube), the participant should be instructed to *talk* through the procedure the first time. The second time through, the participant should not talk, but work as quickly and efficiently as possible to complete the procedure within 20 seconds (from laryngoscope placement through tube insertion). The second time through, only steps 10 through 20 and step 24 need be completed by the participant.

Judge the performance of each step carried out, and check (✔) when the action is completed correctly. If done incorrectly, circle the box so that you can discuss that step later.

Equipment and Supplies

Intubation manikin or other simulation
Laryngoscope with fresh batteries and functioning light source
Blade — No. 1 (fullterm) for use with manikin, or No. 0 if appropriate
ET tubes — 2.5, 3.0, 3.5, 4.0 mm
Stylet
Adhesive tape — 1/2″ or 3/4″ roll
Scissors
Oxygen tubing
Suction device — suction setup with
    10 Fr., or larger, suction catheters
Resuscitation bag and mask
Stethoscope
Shoulder roll

Performance Checklist
Lesson 5—Performing Endotracheal Intubation

Name _____ Instructor _____ Date _____

You will be asked to go through the procedure twice. The first time you should "talk through" the procedure, describing each action or observation made. This is necessary since your instructor is not able to directly view the procedure from insertion of the laryngoscope through placement of the ET tube.

The second time through, you will not need to describe what you are doing. Instead, work as quickly and efficiently as possible to complete the procedure within 20 seconds—from laryngoscope placement through tube insertion. The second time you will not need to prepare the equipment, but you will need to complete steps 10 through 20 and step 24 of this checklist.

Prepares for Intubation   **Instructor:** "The infant weighs _____ grams."

Talk-Through / Demonstration	
	ET Tube
☐	**1. Selects correct size tube**
☐	**2. Cuts tube at 13 cm**
☐	**3. Replaces connector, securing a tight fit**
☐ ☐	**4. Inserts stylet (optional)** • Stylet tip is *within* tip of tube • Secures stylet
	Laryngoscope
☐	**5. Selects appropriate size blade**
☐	**6. Attaches blade to laryngoscope and checks light—replaces batteries or bulb if necessary**
	Additional Equipment
☐	**7. Cuts strip(s) of tape**
☐	**8. Obtains bag and mask** • Bag prepared to give 90–100% O_2 • Bag checked for function • Mask of appropriate size
☐	**9. Obtains or asks for** • Oxygen tubing and source, and • Suction equipment

Performs Intubation

Talk-Through Demonstration	Timed Demonstration	
☐	☐	**10. Correctly positions manikin**
☐	☐	**11. Inserts blade into mouth, holding laryngoscope correctly**
☐	☐	**12. Inserts blade just beyond tongue and lifts using correct motion**
☐	☐	**13. Identifies landmarks seen**
☐	☐	**14. Based upon landmarks seen, takes corrective action if applicable**
☐	☐	**15. Obtains unobstructed view of glottis** (Applies laryngeal pressure, if necessary, using fourth or fifth finger of left hand)
☐	☐	**16. Inserts tube aligning vocal cord guide with vocal cords**
☐	☐	**17. Removes laryngoscope (and stylet if used) while firmly holding tube so that tube position does not change**

		Provides Initial Confirmation of Placement
☐	☐	**18. Manikin:**
		Ventilates
☐	☐	**Correctly states whether tube is properly positioned**
		— or —
☐	☐	**Animal Model:**
		Ventilates and listens to both sides of chest and over abdomen
		Observes chest and abdomen for movement
		Correctly states whether tube is properly positioned
☐	☐	**19. Correctly judges whether corrective action must be taken, and takes the necessary steps if tube is in esophagus or one of the bronchi**
	☐	**20. No more than 20 seconds from blade insertion through correct tube placement**

		Takes Final Steps
☐		**21. States cm marking at level of upper lip**
☐		**22. Tapes tube securely while maintaining proper position**
☐		**23. Shortens tube if more than 4 cm extends from lips**

		Overall
☐	☐	Is gentle in handling infant, laryngoscope, and tube so as to prevent trauma

Appendix:
Endotracheal Suctioning Under Direct Vision

When an infant shows signs of having aspirated meconium, the trachea must be suctioned under direct vision. This involves using a laryngoscope to view the trachea and one of the following for suctioning the trachea:

- ET tube
- Suction catheter, 10 Fr. or larger

The procedures for using each of these two pieces of equipment are given below.

Equipment and Supplies

The equipment and supplies needed for tracheal suctioning are as follows:
- Laryngoscope with appropriate blade (fullterm or premature size)
- ET tube or 10–12 Fr. suction catheter
- Suction setup with tubing

Suctioning Via ET Tube

Suctioning the trachea under direct vision using the *ET tube* is the preferred method for suctioning meconium and may be used for suctioning other material from the trachea as well. This consists of inserting the tube approximately 3 cm below the vocal cords and then applying *continuous* suction as you withdraw the tube. Suction can be applied to the ET tube by use of an adaptor and a regulated wall suction device. Reintubation followed by suctioning may be repeated until the trachea is cleared. The suction pressure should not exceed 100 mm Hg or 4 in Hg.

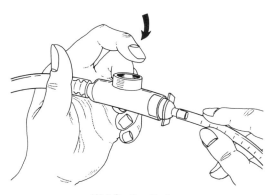

Wall Suction Device

Note:

When suctioning meconium, *do not* attempt to pass a suction catheter *through* an endotracheal tube. You cannot pass a catheter that is large enough to adequately suction the meconium.

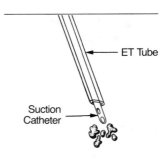

ET Tube

Suction
Catheter

Suction Catheter

The use of a suction catheter and mechanical suctioning device to suction the trachea is a two-person procedure. Under direct vision with a laryngoscope, the operator inserts the suction catheter directly into the trachea and rotates it as it is being withdrawn. The second person provides continuous suction by blocking the catheter's thumb holes as the catheter is being withdrawn.

In directly suctioning the trachea, note the following:

- Suction pressures should not exceed 100 mm Hg or 4 in Hg.

- The suction catheter should have an end hole and side hole (whistle tip) and should be as large as possible—*at least a 10 Fr.*

- The catheter should be rotated and have continuous suction applied as it is being withdrawn. Rotating the catheter facilitates removal of secretions and prevents trauma to the mucosa. Providing continuous suction assures removal of secretions by preventing material clinging to the catheter from falling back into the trachea.

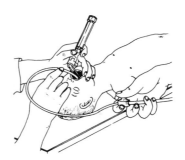

Medications

Lesson 6

Contents

Introduction

Drugs and volume expanders are administered during a resuscitation procedure to:

- Stimulate the heart,
- Increase tissue perfusion, and
- Restore acid-base balance.

Medications may be needed for neonates who do not respond to adequate ventilation with 100% oxygen and chest compressions. The number of medications needed is determined by the infant's condition after the administration of each drug or volume expander.

This lesson will cover the following topics:

- When to begin administering medications,
- What drugs to use in specific circumstances and their anticipated effect, and
- The preparation and administration of each drug and volume expander.

This lesson will teach you the thought process for administering medications during resuscitation. In order for you to carry out this procedure in an actual emergency, the information presented here must be combined with several related skills. For example, some of the skills include:

- Making up appropriate solutions,
- Preparing medications in syringes or I.V. bottles,
- Using commercially prepared prefilled syringes,
- Placing an umbilical venous catheter, and
- Infusing medications through an intravenous line.

Such skills related to administering medications during resuscitation are *not taught* in this lesson.

The dosages in this chapter are based on the infant's weight. In a delivery room, a resuscitation will usually take place before the infant is weighed. Under these circumstances, the weight will have to be estimated from looking at the child and/or from the estimate of the weight prior to delivery.

The pharmacology of the drugs will not be taught. If you desire more information on a given drug, consult a pharmacology reference textbook.

Appendixes

This lesson contains three appendixes that you may find useful.

In the posttest, you will need to calculate dosages for specific infant weights. How to calculate dosages is not taught in the main portion of the lesson. Appendix A contains information on calculating dosages for infants as well as several dosage calculation problems with answers. Refer to Appendix A if you have *any* questions about correctly calculating dosages.

Appendix B contains information on how to prepare and administer dopamine, a drug used in some neonatal settings. Check with your instructor or supervisor as to whether you need to study this information.

The chart in Appendix C contains the important points on preparing and administering each of the medications discussed. As a reference during an emergency, the chart contains a special column with the amounts or dosage of each drug calculated for infants weighing 1, 2, 3, and 4 kg.

Glossary

Below are some key terms and abbreviations used in the lesson. Study these briefly.

E.T. — Endotracheal — given into the trachea via an endotracheal tube.

gm/kg (gram/kilogram) — 1000 grams = one kilogram (e.g., 2500 gm baby weighs 2.5 kg).

Hypovolemia — An abnormally decreased volume of fluid circulating in the bloodstream.

I.M. — Intramuscular.

I.V. — Intravenous.

mcg or μg (microgram) — A microgram (mcg or μg) is 1/1000 of a milligram (mg) — 1000 mcg = 1 mg.

mEq (milliequivalent) — A milliequivalent (mEq) is a unit used to express the amount of a drug in solution.

mL (milliliter) — In dosages, 1 milliliter (mL) and 1 cc are equal amounts — one mL of fluid fills 1 cc of space.

S.Q. — Subcutaneous.

Tissue Perfusion — The flow of blood through the capillary beds of the tissue.

Objectives

The objectives for this lesson are:

- State the specific indication for each of the drugs and volume expanders discussed.
- Identify the major physiological effects of each of the drugs and volume expanders.
- Describe how each drug or volume expander should be prepared, including the recommended concentration of each and the amount that should be prepared for administration.
- State the dosage, route, and rate of administration for each drug and volume expander.
- When given the weight of an infant in grams, calculate the correct dosage of each drug and volume expander.
- Identify the signs of hypovolemia.
- List three volume expanders useful during a neonatal resuscitation.

Decision Table

If . . .	Then . . .
You feel you can pass a test on the objectives . . .	Turn to the posttest.
You wish to know more before trying the posttest . . .	Go on to the next page and begin the lesson.

Routes of Administration

Everyone involved with neonatal resuscitation should be familiar with the available routes of drug administration.

The routes of drug administration include:
- Umbilical vein,
- Peripheral veins,
- Endotracheal instillation.

As you continue on to learn about the individual drugs, you will find that they can *all* be given intravenously, but some drugs can also be administered via the endotracheal tube.

Umbilical Vein

The umbilical vein is the most common vascular route for administering drugs in the delivery room because it can be easily located and cannulated.

Catheter Placement

A 3.5 or 5.0 Fr. umbilical catheter with a single end hole and a radiopaque marker should be used. The catheter should be inserted into the vein of the umbilical stump until the tip of the catheter is just below the skin level, but free flow of blood is present. If the catheter is inserted farther, there is risk of infusing solutions into the liver and possibly causing damage.

Correct	Incorrect
Catheter Just Below Skin Level	Catheter in Too Far

Note:

Consideration should be given to removing the umbilical venous catheter once the resuscitation procedure is over. In the majority of circumstances, if vascular access is desired for continuing care, an umbilical artery or a peripheral vein should be used.

Peripheral Vein

Veins in the scalp and extremities can be used for administering drugs or solutions, but are difficult to access, especially during resuscitation.

Endotracheal Instillation (E.T.)

Some drugs may be injected directly into the bronchial tree via the endotracheal tube. Immediately after the drug is injected, the infant should be given positive-pressure ventilation to distribute the drug deep into the bronchial tree.

Because some of the drug may adhere to the endotracheal tube, some prefer to insert a 5 Fr. feeding tube through the endotracheal tube. The drug is then injected via the feeding tube, which is then flushed with enough normal saline to clear the drug from the feeding tube (0.5 cc for a 15-inch 5 Fr. tube). The feeding tube is then removed and positive-pressure ventilation provided to distribute the drug into the bronchial tree.

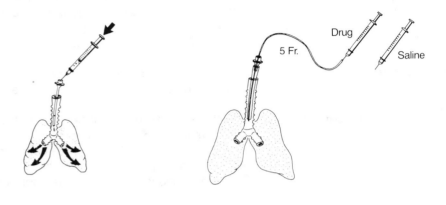

Overview of the Procedure

The majority of infants requiring resuscitation will have a response to prompt and effective ventilation with 100% oxygen. Some will additionally require chest compressions. In those few infants who fail to improve with ventilation and chest compressions, the use of medications becomes necessary. If an infant has no detectable heartbeat, medications should be initiated without delay — at the same time that PPV and chest compressions are started.

Indications for Medications

Thus, medications should be initiated when . . .
- **The infant's heart rate remains below 80 despite adequate ventilation (with 100% oxygen) and chest compressions for a minimum of 30 seconds, or**
- **The heart rate is zero.**

Medications

The medications used during neonatal resuscitation and discussed in this lesson include:

```
Epinephrine
```

| **Volume Expanders** | **Sodium Bicarbonate** |
| For acute bleeding with signs of hypovolemia | For documented or assumed metabolic acidosis |

```
Dopamine
```

Epinephrine, as you will learn, is the first drug administered. If the response to epinephrine is inadequate, a volume expander and/or sodium bicarbonate may be required. The use of each will be discussed.

In a prolonged resuscitative effort in which an infant is in shock and fails to maintain improvement following administration of the above drugs, a dopamine infusion may be established while consultation with a neonatologist is being obtained. Since dopamine is mainly used in an intensive care setting, information about its administration is not included in the main part of the lesson, but can be found in Appendix B.

```
Naloxone Hydrochloride
```

Naloxone hydrochloride (Narcan) is a narcotic antagonist with a very specific use. It may be administered before any other drug, when respiratory depression due to maternal narcotics is suspected.

Medications Not Included

Atropine and calcium are not included in this lesson. Although previously recommended for use in the asphyxiated neonate, there is no current evidence that they are useful in the acute phase of neonatal resuscitation.

Page Layout

A discussion of each drug in this lesson will follow the format shown below. Information related to preparing the medication is presented first, followed by information related to its administration.

Medication
_____

Introduction

_____

**Indications
For Use**

_____

Preparation

    Recommended
    Concentration

    Preparing
    Syringe

_____

Administration

    Dosage

    Route

    Rate

    Effects

    Anticipated
    Signs

    Follow-up

_____

Preparation Section

In the "Preparation" section you will learn:
- The *concentration* of the drug you should administer, and
- A recommended *amount* of the drug you should draw into a syringe, in anticipation of need.

The recommended amount of a drug that should be made ready is based on the amount required by a fullterm infant. The actual amount that is administered is decided by the individual in charge of the resuscitation.

If delivery of an asphyxiated, volume-depleted, or drug-depressed infant is anticipated, management is facilitated if drugs are prepared *prior* to the delivery. Advantages of preparing drugs ahead of time include:
- There is no delay in administering medications,
- All staff members are free to participate in the resuscitation effort, and
- Chances of a medication error are reduced when drugs are not prepared under pressure.

Simplify Preparation

All of the drugs discussed in this lesson (except dopamine) are commercially available in the concentrations recommended and in small volumes specifically designed for neonatal use. In some circumstances, they are available in prefilled syringes. Your pharmacy should be requested to supply these neonatal preparations for use in the delivery room and nursery. To do so will save time and money and reduce medication errors.

Know Your Stock

Before completing this lesson, be sure you are fully aware of the drugs currently stocked on your unit for use with neonates requiring resuscitation. For each medication, know the concentration and how it is packaged.

Administration Section

The "Administration" section for each drug will familiarize you with the:
- Dosage/kg — sometimes expressed as a range,
- Acceptable route(s) for administering the medication,
- Rate of administration,
- Basic effects of the medication,
- Anticipated signs to observe in the neonate, and
- Follow-up action.

Reference Chart

Appendix C contains a chart with important points on preparing and administering each of the medications discussed. You may find it useful to copy and keep it near the area where medications are prepared.

Epinephrine

Epinephrine hydrochloride (sometimes referred to as adrenaline chloride) is a cardiac stimulant. Epinephrine increases the strength and rate of cardiac contractions.

Indications For Use

Epinephrine should be administered when:
- **Heart rate remains below 80 per minute despite a minimum of 30 seconds of adequate ventilation with 100% oxygen *and* chest compressions, or**
- **Heart rate is zero.** If a heartbeat cannot be detected, epinephrine should be given immediately—at the same time PPV and chest compressions are initiated.

Preparation

Recommended Concentration

> 1:10,000

(Epinephrine is commercially available in a 1:10,000 concentration, eliminating the need to dilute the 1:1,000 concentration.)

Preparing Syringe

> Prepare 1 mL in a syringe

Administration

Dosage

> 0.1–0.3 mL/kg of the 1:10,000 solution

Route

> Intravenously (I.V.) or per endotracheal tube (E.T.)

When given E.T.: To aid delivery of the small amount of drug required, the epinephrine may be diluted 1:1 with normal saline.

Rate

> Give rapidly

Effects

- Increases strength and rate of cardiac contractions.
- Causes peripheral vasoconstriction.

Anticipated Signs

Heart rate should rise to 100 or above within 30 seconds after infusion.

Follow-up

- **If heart rate remains below 100,** consider:
  - *Epinephrine (*readministered)—may be repeated every 5 minutes if required,
  - *Volume expander*—if there is evidence of acute blood loss with signs of hypovolemia,
  - Sodium bicarbonate—with a documented or assumed metabolic acidosis.

Review 1

Below is a summary of the conditions under which medications should be initiated during resuscitation. The flow diagram shows the drugs to be used.

When to Begin

During resuscitation, medications should be initiated if:

• Heart rate is zero, or

• Heart rate remains below 80 per minute *after* at least 30 seconds of ventilation with 100% oxygen and chest compressions.

Flow Diagram

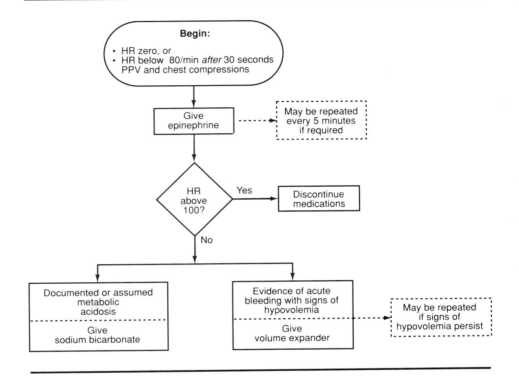

Chart

Medication	Concentration To Administer	Preparation	Dosage/ Route	Rate/Precautions
Epinephrine	1:10,000	1 mL	0.1–0.3 mL/kg I.V. or E.T.	Give rapidly May dilute 1:1 with normal saline if giving E.T.

Practice Activity 1

Follow the directions for each of the items below.

Fill In

1–2. Under what two circumstances would you initiate administering medications during resuscitation?

- _____
  _____

- _____
  _____

What is the correct concentration of epinephrine, and what amount should be drawn up in a syringe?

3. Concentration: _____.

4. Amount to prepare: _____

Write the correct dosage, route, and rate of administration for epinephrine.

5. Dosage: _____

6. Route(s) of administration: _____

7. Rate of administration: _____

8–10. If after the initial administration of epinephrine the heart rate remains below 100, what three medications might you consider giving?

- _____

- _____

- _____

Multiple Choice

11–12. What are the two *major* effects of epinephrine?

_____
A. Increases tissue perfusion
B. Causes peripheral vasoconstriction
C. Increases strength and rate of cardiac contractions
D. Corrects metabolic acidosis

Practice Activity 1: Answers

The answers for the practice activity are given below. Be sure and review the material for any questions that you miss.

Fill In

1–2. • Heart rate is zero, or
  • Heart rate is below 80 after 30 seconds of PPV (with 100% oxygen) and chest compressions

3. Concentration: 1:10,000

4. Preparation: 1 mL in a syringe

5. Dosage: 0.1—0.3 mL/kg (of 1:10,000 solution)

6. Routes: I.V. or E.T.

7. Rate: Give rapidly

8–10. • Epinephrine (readministered)
  • Volume expander
  • Sodium bicarbonate

Multiple Choice

11–12. B, C

Decision Table

If . . .	Then . . .
You correctly answered 11 of the 12 items . . .	Well done. Continue with the next page.
You were correct on fewer than 11 items . . .	Review the material for the questions you missed, then go on to the next section of the lesson.

Volume Expanders

Volume expanders are used to counteract the effects of hypovolemia by increasing vascular volume and subsequently tissue perfusion.

Hypovolemia should be considered in *any* infant who requires resuscitation. It occurs more frequently in the newly born infant than is commonly recognized.

Signs of Hypovolemia

It is important to be aware of the signs of hypovolemia, since blood loss by the infant is frequently not obvious.

An infant may suffer a 10–15% loss of total blood volume and demonstrate no more than a slight decrease in systolic blood pressure—usually not perceived in the delivery room. A 20% or greater loss in total blood volume results in the following signs:

- Pallor persisting after oxygenation
- Weak pulses with a *good* heart rate
- Poor response to resuscitative efforts
- Decreased blood pressure (may not be available)

Note:

In acute blood loss, determination of Hgb and Hct are misleading since the values may initially be normal.

Indication for Use

A volume expander is indicated during resuscitation when there is:
- **Evidence of acute bleeding with signs of hypovolemia.**

Types of Volume Expanders

Four volume expanders may be administered. The four most commonly used volume expanders are:

- Whole blood (O-negative blood cross-matched with the mother's blood)

- 5% albumin/saline solution (or other plasma substitute)

- Normal saline

- Ringer's lactate

Although compatible whole blood is the best volume expander, it may be difficult to obtain on a practical basis.

Preparation

Be aware of how each of the volume expanders is packaged in your institution and how each might need to be prepared for administration. Some will require use of a filter.

Prepare Syringe or Drip System

Draw 40 mL into a syringe or infusion set

Administration

Dosage

| 10 mL/kg |

Route

| I.V. |

Rate

| Give over 5–10 minutes |

Effects

- Increases vascular volume
- Decreases metabolic acidosis by increasing tissue perfusion

Anticipated Signs

Blood pressure should increase, pulses become stronger, and pallor improve.

Follow-up

- May be repeated if signs of hypovolemia persist.
- With little or no improvement:
  - Consider the presence of metabolic acidosis and need for sodium bicarbonate.
  - With a persistent decrease in blood pressure, consider use of dopamine.

Review 2

Below is a summary of the important information related to the use of volume expanders and a cumulative chart of the two drugs discussed so far.

Indication

When there is evidence of acute bleeding with signs of hypovolemia, a volume expander is indicated.

Signs of Hypovolemia

The signs of hypovolemia are:
• Pallor persisting after oxygenation
• Weak pulses with a *good* heart rate
• Poor response to resuscitative efforts
• Decreased blood pressure

Chart

Medication	Concentration to Administer	Preparation	Dosage/ Route	Rate/Precautions
Epinephrine	1:10,000	1 mL	0.1–0.3 mL/kg I.V. or E.T.	Give rapidly May dilute 1:1 with normal saline if giving E.T.
Volume Expanders	Whole Blood 5% Albumin Normal Saline Ringer's Lactate	40 mL	10 mL/kg I.V.	Give over 5–10 min Give by syringe or I.V. drip

Practice Activity 2

In this practice activity you will be asked to recall information related to the use of volume expanders during resuscitation.

Fill In

1–4. List the four volume expanders that might be used during neonatal resuscitation.

- _____
- _____
- _____
- _____

5. State the indication given for using a volume expander.

_____

_____

6. How much should be drawn up in preparation for administration? _____

Write the correct dosage, route, and rate of administration.

7. Dosage: _____

8. Route: _____

9. Rate: _____

Selection

Which of the following are signs of hypovolemia?

10–13. _____
A. Pallor persisting after oxygenation
B. Weak pulses with a good heart rate
C. Elevated blood pressure
D. Poor response to resuscitation
E. Bounding pulses with normal heart rate
F. Decreased blood pressure

Identify effects of the following medications.

Effects

14–16. Epinephrine
A. Decreases metabolic acidosis by increasing tissue perfusion

_____
B. Increases the heart rate

17–18. Volume Expander
C. Causes peripheral vasoconstriction
D. Increases vascular volume

_____
E. Increases strength of cardiac contractions

True/False

Identify each of the following as "true" or "false."

19. _____ A normal hematocrit in an infant requiring resuscitation rules out hypovolemia.

20. _____ Infants experiencing a 5–10% loss of total blood volume will have obvious signs of hypovolemia.

21. _____ Hypovolemia should be considered in any infant requiring resuscitation.

Practice Activity 2: Answers

Check your answers against those given here.

Fill In

1–4. (In any order)
- Whole Blood
- 5% albumin
- Normal saline
- Ringer's lactate

5. Evidence of acute bleeding with signs of hypovolemia.
6. Amount to prepare: 40 mL
7. Dosage: 10 mL/kg
8. Route: I.V.
9. Rate: Give over 5–10 minutes

Selection

10–13. A, B, D, F

14–16. B, C, E

17–18. A, D,

True/False

19. False — In acute blood loss, the Hct remains normal for a period of time following the episode.

20. False — Signs of blood loss are often not obvious in an infant until an infant has lost 20–25% of total blood volume.

21. True

Decision

If . . .	Then . . .
You answered all questions correctly or missed no more than 2 . . .	Excellent. Once you have reviewed the correct answers for items you missed, continue.
You were incorrect on more than 2 questions . . .	Carefully review the section on volume expanders.

Sodium Bicarbonate

During prolonged asphyxia, diminished tissue oxygenation leads to a build-up of lactic acid, which results in metabolic acidosis. The progression of acidosis should be *slowed* by assuring oxygenation of the blood, elimination of carbon dioxide, and adequate tissue perfusion. To *correct* the existing acidosis in an infant who has not responded to this point, sodium bicarbonate may be administered when ventilation is adequate.

Indication for Use

Sodium bicarbonate is indicated when there is:
- **Documented or assumed metabolic acidosis.**

Note:

Sodium bicarbonate should only be used after ventilation is established.

Preparation

Recommended Concentration

> 0.5 mEq/mL = 4.2% Solution

4.2% sodium bicarbonate is commercially available in prefilled 10-mL syringes.

Preparing Syringe

> Draw 20 mL sodium bicarbonate into a syringe
> *or*
> Prepare 2 10-mL prefilled syringes

Administration

Dosage

> 2 mEq/kg

Route

> I.V.

Rate

> Give slowly—over at least 2 minutes
> (1 mEq/kg/minute)

Effects

- Corrects metabolic acidosis by raising the pH of the blood, and
- Provides some volume expansion resulting from the hypertonic solution of sodium.

Anticipated Signs

Heart rate should rise to 100 or above within 30 seconds after infusion is completed.

Follow-up

Heart rate below 100: Consider readministration of epinephrine and continue with volume expanders, ventilation, and chest compressions. If persistent hypotension is present, consider administration of dopamine.

Caution:

- Effective ventilation must *precede* and *accompany* the administration of sodium bicarbonate.
- To minimize the risk of intraventricular hemorrhage, administer sodium bicarbonate using the concentration and rate recommended.
- Sodium bicarbonate may be useful in a prolonged resuscitation to help correct a metabolic acidosis that has been documented or is assumed to be present, but its use is discouraged in brief arrests or episodes of bradycardia.

Review 3

A review of the information related to the use of sodium bicarbonate is presented here.

Indication

When there is a metabolic acidosis that has been documented or is assumed to be present, sodium bicarbonate may be used.

Precautions

Effective ventilation must precede and accompany the administration of sodium bicarbonate.

The risk of intraventricular hemorrhage may be decreased if:

• A 4.2% (0.5 mEq/mL) solution of sodium bicarbonate is used, and

• If the drug is administered slowly—at least over 2 minutes.

Chart

Medication	Concentration to Administer	Preparation	Dosage/ Route	Rate/Precautions
Epinephrine	1:10,000	1 mL	0.1–0.3 mL/kg I.V. or E.T.	Give rapidly May dilute 1:1 with normal saline if giving E.T.
Volume Expanders	Whole Blood 5% Albumin Normal Saline Ringer's Lactate	40 mL	10 mL/kg I.V.	Give over 5–10 min Give by syringe or I.V. drip
Sodium Bicarbonate	0.5 mEq/mL (4.2% solution)	20 mL or two 10-mL prefilled syringes	2 mEq/kg I.V.	Give *slowly,* over at least 2 min Give only if infant being effectively ventilated

Practice Activity 3

The questions below will test your understanding of the proper use of sodium bicarbonate during resuscitation.

Fill In

1. State the indications for use.

   _____

2. Recommended concentration: _____

3. Amount to draw up or have available: _____

4. Dosage: _____

5. Route: _____

6. Rate: _____

7–8. State two precautions in administering sodium bicarbonate to decrease the risk of an intraventricular hemorrhage.

   • _____

   • _____

Multiple Choice

Identify the major effect(s) of the drugs listed.

9–10. Sodium Bicarbonate

_____

11–12. Volume Expander

_____

13–14. Epinephrine

_____

Effects

A. Increases strength and rate of cardiac contractions
B. Is a narcotic antagonist
C. Increases vascular volume
D. Corrects metabolic acidosis by raising the pH of the blood
E. Causes peripheral vasoconstriction
F. Helps correct metabolic acidosis by increasing tissue perfusion
G. Provides some volume expansion resulting from the hypertonic solution of sodium.

Practice Activity 3: Answers

Compare your answers with those given below.

Fill In

1. Documented or assumed metabolic acidosis

2. Concentration: 0.5 mEq/mL or 4.2%

3. Prepare: 20 mL (either in one syringe or two 10-mL prefilled syringes)

4. Dosage: 2 mEq/kg

5. Route: I.V.

6. Rate: Give slowly over at least 2 minutes

7–8. • Administer recommended concentration (4.2% or 0.5 mEq/mL solution)
   • Give slowly, over 2 minutes

Multiple Choice

9–10. **D, G** (**C** and **F** could also be considered correct)

11–12. **C, F**

13–14. **A, E**

Decision

If . . .	Then . . .
You had all the answers correct or missed no more than 2 . . .	Continue to learn about Narcan.
You were correct on fewer than 12 of the 14 questions . . .	Review this section carefully. Discuss with your instructor any questions you may have.

Naloxone Hydrochloride

Naloxone hydrochloride, commonly known as Narcan*, is a narcotic antagonist that reverses respiratory depression induced by a variety of narcotics. In the neonate, the depression of respirations by narcotics most commonly occurs when narcotics are administered to the mother within 4 hours of delivery.

It is important that the infant with depressed respiratory effort due to maternal narcotics receive prompt and adequate ventilatory assistance until naloxone can be administered and exert its effect. If timely and effective ventilation is provided, the infant should not suffer asphyxia, and additional resuscitative measures will not be necessary.

Indications for Use

Naloxone is indicated when there is:

Severe respiratory depression,

> *AND*

A history of maternal narcotic administration within the past 4 hours.

Preparation

Concentration

> 0.4 mg/mL or 1.0 mg/mL solution

Prepare

> 1 mL in a syringe

Administration

Dosage

> **0.1 mg/kg**

Routes

> E.T., I.V. — Preferred
> I.M., S.Q. — Acceptable
>   Delayed onset of action

Rate

> Inject rapidly

Effects

Narcotic antagonist

Signs

Spontaneous respirations

Follow-up

Monitor respirations and heart rate closely; readminister naloxone if respiratory depression recurs.

Note:

The duration of action of naloxone is 1–4 hours. The duration of action of the narcotic may exceed that of the naloxone, necessitating repeated doses of naloxone.

Be aware that the administration of naloxone to an infant of a narcotic-addicted mother may result in severe seizures.

*Narcan is a trademark of Du Pont Pharmaceuticals.

Review 4

Below is information related to naloxone.

**Indication
For Naloxone**

Naloxone is indicated when there is:
- Depressed respirations in the newborn,
    and
- A history of maternal narcotic administration within the past 4 hours.

Chart

Medication	Concentration to Administer	Preparation	Dosage	Rate/Route
Naloxone	0.4 mg/mL	1 mL	0.1 mg/kg (0.25 mL/kg)	Give rapidly I.V., E.T. preferred I.M., S.Q. acceptable
	1.0 mg/mL	1 mL	0.1 mg/kg (0.1 mL/kg)	

Practice Activity 4

This practice activity will test your knowledge of naloxone.

Completion

1. Describe the indication for naloxone during a neonatal resuscitation.

(Neonate's condition:) _____

_____ *and*

(Maternal history:) _____

_____

State the following for naloxone injection:

2. Two recommended concentrations: _____ and _____

3. Preparation: _____

4. Dosage: _____

5–8. Routes: _____

9. Rate of administration: _____

True/False

10. _____ In infants with respiratory depression due to maternal narcotics, naloxone eliminates the need to initiate positive-pressure ventilation.

11. _____ The duration of action of naloxone may be less than that of the narcotic, necessitating repeated doses of naloxone.

12. _____ Infants with depressed respiratory effort due to narcotics will all undergo some degree of asphyxia, although it may be mild.

Practice Activity 4: Answers

Check your answers with those given below.

Completion

1. • Neonate's condition: Infant has respiratory depression.

   and

   • Maternal history: There is a history of maternal narcotic administration within the past 4 hours.

2. Concentrations: 0.4 mg/mL and 1.0 mg/mL

3. Preparation: 1 mL in a syringe

4. Dosage: 0.1 mg/kg

5–8. Routes: I.V., E.T., S.Q., I.M.

9. Rate: Give rapidly

True/False

10. **False** — With respiratory depression, PPV should be provided until the naloxone can exert its effect.

11. **True**

12. **False** — There should be no asphyxia if effective ventilation is provided promptly and continued until naloxone can exert its effect.

Decision

If . . .	Then . . .
You had all the answers correct or missed no more than 1 . . .	Continue to the next lesson.
You were correct on fewer than 11 of the 12 questions . . .	Review this section carefully. Discuss with your instructor any questions you may have.

Summary

This summary contains key points related to the use of medications during neonatal resuscitation.

Medications
 Epinephrine
 Volume Expander
 Sodium
  Bicarbonate

Dopamine

Naloxone Hydrochloride

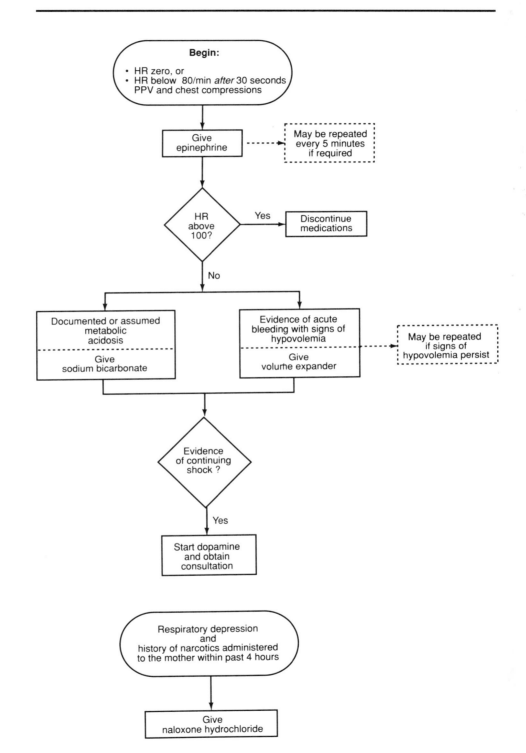

Signs of Hypovolemia

The signs of hypovolemia are:
- Pallor persisting despite oxygenation
- Weak pulses with a *good* heart rate
- Poor response to resuscitative efforts
- Decreased blood pressure

Routes of Administration

The most common route for administering drugs or volume expanders in the delivery room is the umbilical vein. Alternative routes may be used for epinephrine and naloxone hydrochloride. The routes that may be used for the medications discussed are shown in the following chart.

Medications	Routes		
	I.V.	E.T.	Other
Epinephrine	X	X	
Volume Expander	X		
Sodium Bicarbonate	X		
Naloxone Hydrochloride	X	X	I.M., S.Q. Delayed onset of action

Rates of Administration

Rates for administering the medications used during neonatal resuscitation vary. To prevent complications and maximize the therapeutic effect, use the following rates.

Medications	Rates
Epinephrine	Give rapidly
Volume Expander	Give over 5–10 minutes
Sodium Bicarbonate	Give slowly, over at least 2 minutes
Naloxone Hydrochloride	Give rapidly

Chart

Medication	Concentration to Administer	Preparation	Dosage/ Route	Rate/Precautions
Epinephrine	1:10,000	1 mL	0.1–0.3 mL/kg I.V. or E.T.	Give rapidly May dilute 1:1 with normal saline if giving E.T.
Volume Expanders	Whole Blood 5% Albumin Normal Saline Ringer's Lactate	40 mL	10 mL/kg I.V.	Give over 5–10 min Give by syringe or I.V. drip
Sodium Bicarbonate	0.5 mEq/mL (4.2% solution)	20 mL or two 10-mL prefilled syringes	2 mEq/kg I.V.	Give *slowly,* over at least 2 min Give only if infant being effectively ventilated
Naloxone	0.4 mg/mL	1 mL	0.1 mg/kg (0.25 mL/kg) I.V., E.T., I.M., S.Q.	Give rapidly I.V., E.T. preferred I.M., S.Q. acceptable
	1.0 mg/mL	1 mL	0.1 mg/kg (0.1 mL/kg) I.V., E.T., I.M., S.Q.	

Practice Activity 5

This last practice activity will test your knowledge of all of the medications discussed previously.

Fill In

For each of the medications below, state the recommended dosage and the amount of the drug appropriate for an infant of the specified weight.

Calculate infant's weight to the *nearest* tenth of a kg. For example, 1570 gm = 1.57 kg = 1.6 kg (when rounded to nearest tenth of a kg). See Appendix A if you have any difficulty calculating the dosages.

Volume Expander

1. Recommended dosage: _____

2. Dose for 1230-gm infant: _____

Epinephrine

3. Recommended dosage: _____

4. Dosage range for 3700-gm infant: _____

Sodium Bicarbonate

5. Recommended dosage: _____

6. Dose for 2280-gm infant: _____

Designate the route(s) and rate for administering each medication by completing the following chart. In the "I.V." and "E.T." columns, use a check (✔) to indicate the appropriate route. If routes other than "I.V" or "E.T." are appropriate, write them in the "Other" column.

7–18.

Medications	Routes			Rate of Administration
	I.V.	E.T.	Other	
Epinephrine				
Volume Expander				
Sodium Bicarbonate				
Naloxone Hydrochloride				

Matching

19–25. Match items in the "Effects" column with the appropriate drug or volume expander.

Drug or Volume Expander

_____ Epinephrine

_____ Volume Expander

_____ Sodium Bicarbonate

_____ Naloxone Hydrochloride

Effects

A. Decreases metabolic acidosis by increasing tissue perfusion

B. Is a narcotic antagonist

C. Provides some volume expansion resulting from the hypertonic solution of sodium

D. Increases vascular volume

E. Increases the rate and strength of cardiac contractions

F. Corrects metabolic acidosis by raising the pH of the blood

G. Causes peripheral vasoconstriction

Match the recommended concentration(s) with each drug or volume expander. Place the letter preceding the concentration (Column B) in the space beside the medication in Column A.

Column A — Medication

_____ **26.** Epinephrine

_____ **27.** Albumin

_____ **28.** Sodium Bicarbonate

_____ **29.**
_____ **30.** } Naloxone Hydrochloride

Column B — Concentration

A. 5% solution

B. 0.4 mg/mL

C. 0.5 mEq/mL

D. 1:10,000

E. 25% solution

F. 1 mEq/mL

G. 1.0 mg/mL

H. 1:1000

Select the correct preparation of each drug and volume expander. Place the letter preceding the preparation in the space beside the drug or volume expander in Column A. You may use items in Column B more than once.

Column A — Medication

_____ **31.** Epinephrine

_____ **32.** Naloxone Hydrochloride

_____ **33.** Sodium Bicarbonate

_____ **34.** Volume Expander

Column B — Preparation

A. 1 mL in a syringe

B. 20 mL in a syringe, or 2 10-mL prefilled syringes

C. 40 mL to be given by syringe or drip

D. 5 mL in a syringe

E. 2 mL in a syringe

Case Situations

Imagine yourself in each of the situations below. Indicate which medication (drug or a volume expander) should be administered in each case.

35. A neonate has been receiving ventilation with 100% oxygen and chest compressions for a minimum of 30 seconds. The heart rate is 50. What drug should be given in this situation?

_____

36–38. If the infant's heart rate was 70/minute after receiving the drug identified in Question 35, what three medications might you consider giving?

- _____

- _____

- _____

Practice Activity 5: Answers

Compare your answers with those given below.

Fill In

Volume Expander

1. Dosage: 10 mL/kg

2. Dose for 1230-gm (1.2-kg) infant: 12 mL

Epinephrine

3. Dosage: 0.1–0.3 mL/kg

4. Dosage range for 3700-gm (3.7-kg) infant: .37 to 1.11 mL

Sodium Bicarbonate

5. Dosage: 2 mEq/kg

6. Dose for 2280-gm (2.3-kg) infant: 4.6 mEq or 9.2 mL

7–18.

Medications	Routes			Rate of Administration
	I.V.	**E.T.**	**Other**	
Epinephrine	✔	✔		Give rapidly
Volume Expander	✔			Give over 5–10 min.
Sodium Bicarbonate	✔			Give slowly, over at least 2 min.
Naloxone Hydrochloride	✔	✔	S.Q., I.M.	Give rapidly

Matching

19–25. **E, G** Epinephrine

A, D Volume expander

C, F Sodium bicarbonate (**A** and **D** may be considered correct)

B Naloxone hydrochloride

26. D

27. A

28. C

29–30. B, G

31. A

32. A

33. B

34. C

Case Situations

35. Epinephrine

36–38. • Epinephrine (readministered)
   • Volume expander
   • Sodium bicarbonate

Decision

If . . .	Then . . .
You had them all correct or missed no more than 4 . . .	Go on to the posttest.
You missed 5 or more . . .	Study the sections of the book you need to review. Also carefully review the summary before taking the posttest.

Posttest
Lesson 6 — Medications

Name _____   Date _____

All of the following relate to the four medications presented. Complete each item; be sure to include the correct unit of measurement when appropriate, e.g., mg, mEq, mL, %.

To successfully complete this posttest you must correctly answer *all* questions preceded by a * and miss no more than two of the other items.

Epinephrine

*1–2. Describe the two situations in which epinephrine should be initiated during resuscitation.

- _____

_____

- _____

_____

What is the correct concentration, amount drawn up in a syringe, and dosage of epinephrine?

*3. Concentration: _____

4. Amount to prepare: _____

*5. Dosage: _____

*6. A 2300-gm infant who is being resuscitated requires epinephrine. What dosage should be administered? _____
(Use space below for calculations.)

*7. What route or routes might be used? _____

8. State the correct rate of administration. _____

9. If required, how often can epinephrine be readministered?

_____

*10. If the heart rate remains below 100, what three medications might you consider giving?

- _____
- _____
- _____

Volume Expanders

*11. When is a volume expander indicated during resuscitation?

_____

_____

12. List at least three volume expanders that may be used for neonates in the delivery room.

- _____
- _____
- _____

13. Mrs. Allen is undergoing an emergency cesarean section because of an abruptio placenta. In preparing medications that might be needed for the infant, how much of a volume expander would you prepare?

_____

*14. State the dosage for a volume expander. _____

*15. The need for a volume expander for baby Allen is apparent. She weighs approximately 2800 gm. How much would you administer?

_____

*16. What route or routes might you use? _____

*17. How rapidly would you administer the volume expander? _____

Which of the following are signs of hypovolemia?

18–21. _____
- **A.** Poor response to resuscitation
- **B.** Normal blood pressure
- **C.** Pallor persisting after oxygenation
- **D.** Central cyanosis
- **E.** Weak pulses with a good heart rate
- **F.** Decreased blood pressure
- **G.** Bounding pulses with a good heart rate

Sodium Bicarbonate

*22. When, during resuscitation, is sodium bicarbonate indicated?

_____

Write the correct concentration and volume to prepare of sodium bicarbonate.

*23. Concentration: _____

*24. Amount to prepare: _____

*25. What is the dosage for sodium bicarbonate? _____

*26. Baby Johnson is a 4680-gm infant whose mother is a diabetic. After a difficult delivery, resuscitation is necessary. Sodium bicarbonate is now indicated. How much should be administered? _____

*27. What route or routes should be used? _____

*28. How rapidly should sodium bicarbonate be given? _____

Naloxone Hydrochloride

*29. Describe the indication for naloxone hydrochloride during a neonatal resuscitation.

(Neonate's condition:) _____

_____ and

(Maternal history:) _____

_____

State the following for naloxone:

*30. Two concentrations recommended for administration: _____ and _____

*31. Amount to prepare: _____

*32. Routes to administer: _____

*33. Rate of administration: _____

*34. Dosage: _____

*35. Mrs. Thomas was given 50 mg of Demerol at 9:30 a.m. At 10:45, her membranes ruptured, and 15 minutes later she delivered a 3230-gm infant. At birth, the baby had an excellent heart rate but *very poor* respiratory effort. PPV was initiated and naloxone was ordered. Calculate how many milligrams are an appropriate dose for this baby. _____

Major Effects

36–42. Identify the *major* effects of each drug and volume expander.

Drug or Volume Expander	Effects
_____ Epinephrine	**A.** Causes peripheral vasoconstriction
	B. Is a narcotic antagonist
_____ Volume Expander	**C.** Provides some volume expansion resulting from the hypertonic solution of sodium
	D. Increases vascular volume
_____ Sodium Bicarbonate	**E.** Increases the rate and strength of cardiac contractions
	F. Corrects metabolic acidosis by raising the pH of the blood
_____ Naloxone Hydrochloride	**G.** Decreases metabolic acidosis by increasing tissue perfusion

Lesson 6 Posttest: Answers

Carefully check your answers against those given below.

Epinephrine

1–2. • Heart rate is zero, or
- Heart rate is below 80 after 30 seconds of PPV (with 100% oxygen) and chest compressions

3. Concentration: 1:10,000

4. Prepare: 1 mL in a syringe

5. Dosage: 0.1–0.3 mL/kg

6. Dosage range for 2.3-kg baby: .23–.69 mL

7. Routes: I.V. or E.T.

8. Rate: Give rapidly

9. Every 5 minutes

10. • Epinephrine (readministered)
- Volume expander
- Sodium bicarbonate

Volume Expander

11. When there is evidence of acute blood loss with signs of hypovolemia

12. (Any three of the following)
- Whole blood
- 5% albumin/saline solution
- Normal saline
- Ringer's lactate

13. Prepare: 40 mL

14. Dosage: 10 mL/kg

15. Dose for 2.8-kg baby: 28 mL

16. Route: I.V.

17. Rate: Give over 5–10 minutes

18–21. A, C, E, F

Sodium Bicarbonate

22. When there is a metabolic acidosis that has been documented or is assumed

23. Concentration: 0.5 mEq/mL or 4.2% solution

24. Prepare: 20 mL or two 10-mL prefilled syringes

25. Dosage: 2 mEq/kg

26. Dosage for a 4.7-kg baby: 9.4 mEq or 18.8 mL

27. Route: I.V.

28. Rate: Give over at least 2 minutes
       (1 mEq/kg/min)

Naloxone Hydrochloride

29. • Neonate's condition: Infant has respiratory depression

and

   • Maternal history: There is a history of maternal narcotic administration within the past 4 hours

30. Concentrations: 0.4 mg/mL and 1.0 mg/mL

31. Prepare: 1 mL

32. Routes: I.V., E.T., S.Q., I.M.

33. Rate: Give rapidly

34. Dosage: 0.1 mg/kg

35. Dosage for a 3.2-kg baby: 0.32 mg

Major Effects

36–42. A, E Epinephrine

D, G Volume Expander

C, F Sodium Bicarbonate (**D** and **G** are also acceptable answers)

B   Naloxone Hydrochloride

Decision

If ...	Then ...
You were correct on *all* items, or you successfully answered all questions preceded by a * and missed no more than 2 others ...	You've done very well completing a difficult and important lesson.
You missed any item preceded by a * or missed more than 2 others ...	Study the text content for any questions you missed, then try the posttest again. See your instructor if you have any questions.

Appendix A: Calculating Dosages

Correct calculation of medication doses is critical for the safe care of neonates. You will be called upon to calculate dosages for specific infant weights in the posttest. If you have any questions about your ability to do so correctly, or if you would like a review of calculating dosages, study this section.

Calculations

When calculating drug dosages, it is sufficient to use the infant's weight **to the nearest tenth of a kilogram.** For instance, if an infant's weight is known to be 2835 gm, the weight converted to kilograms is 2.835 kg. The weight to use in calculating the drug dose is to the **nearest** tenth of a kilogram (2.8 kg in this case). If the weight is 2865 gm, you would round it off to 2.9 kg.

Example 1

An infant weighs 3140 gm. You have decided that sodium bicarbonate is needed. The dose is 2 mEq/kg.

3140 gm = 3.14 kg. Rounded to the nearest tenth of a kilogram, that would be 3.1 kg.

2 mEq × 3.1 kg = 6.2 mEq or 12.4 mL (of a 0.5 mEq/mL solution).

Example 2

An infant weighs 2470 gm and requires epinephrine. The dose is 0.1–0.3-mL/kg. Since the dose of epinephrine is expressed as a range, you would need to calculate the dosage for both 0.1 mL/kg and 0.3 mL/kg.

2470 gm = 2.5 kg (rounded to the nearest tenth of a kg)

2.5 kg × 0.1 mL = 0.25 mL

2.5 kg × 0.3 mL = 0.75 mL

The dose range for this infant would be 0.25 mL–0.75 mL.

Practice

Below you will find four dosage calculation problems. As you work through them, remember these points:
• Use kg weight to the *nearest tenth of a kg.*
• Be sure you place the decimal point correctly.
• Be sure to include the correct unit of measurement, e.g., mg, mEq, mL.
• Recheck your multiplication to avoid errors.

Write your answer in the space provided. Use the area beneath each question for your calculations.

You should have studied the medications taught in this lesson before attempting these problems, since you will need to know the correct dosage for each of the medications.

Problem 1   You have decided that a 2160-gm infant should be given a volume expander. How much should be administered?

Problem 2   A 2510-gm infant needs sodium bicarbonate. What dosage is appropriate?

Problem 3   An infant requires naloxone hydrochloride. He weighs 3410 gm. How many milligrams are appropriate for the infant?

Problem 4   A 910-gm infant requires epinephrine. What dosage range is appropriate?

Answers

Here are the answers and calculations for the preceding problems.

Problem 1

2160 gm = 2.2 kg
dosage of volume expander is 10 mL/kg

10 mL × 2.2 = 22 mL

Problem 2

2510 gm = 2.5 kg
dosage of sodium bicarbonate is 2 mEq/kg

2 mEq × 2.5 = 5 mEq or 10 mL of a 4.2% (0.5 mEq/mL) solution

Problem 3

3410 gm = 3.4 kg
dosage of naloxone hydrochloride is 0.1 mg/kg

0.1 mg × 3.4 = 0.34 mg

Problem 4

910 gm = .9 kg
dosage of epinephrine is 0.1–0.3 mL/kg

0.1 mL × .9 = .09 mL

0.3 mL × .9 = .27 mL

.09 mL–.27 mL

How Did You Do?

If you had trouble with these calculations, try to pinpoint the source of error.
- Using the wrong numbers in computing dosage, for example:
  - Incorrect kg weight, or
  - Incorrect dosage/kg
- Decimal point error (right numbers, but decimal point in wrong spot)
- Multiplication error resulting in incorrect numbers
- Using an incorrect unit of measurement (mg instead of mEq)

Ask your instructor for assistance if you had difficulty with these problems.

Appendix B: Dopamine Hydrochloride

One of the effects of asphyxia is to decrease cardiac contractility with a consequent decrease in cardiac output. If an infant undergoes a prolonged resuscitation, including administration of epinephrine, a volume expander, and sodium bicarbonate, and continues to have poor peripheral perfusion, thready pulses, and evidence of shock, a dopamine infusion may help raise the blood pressure.

Dopamine hydrochloride has the primary effect of strengthening cardiac contractions, thereby increasing cardiac output and ultimately raising the neonate's blood pressure.

If it has not been obtained to this point, the institution of dopamine should mark the point at which it is imperative that consultation with a neonatologist or referral nursery be sought for guidance about the continuing care of a very sick neonate.

Additional Considerations

The administration of dopamine has some additional considerations. It must be given as a continuous infusion with the flow rate carefully controlled with an infusion pump. Since dopamine affects cardiac output and blood pressure, the infant receiving dopamine requires *continuous monitoring* and frequent assessment of heart rate and blood pressure.

Indications for Use

After giving epinephrine, a volume expander, and sodium bicarbonate, administer dopamine if:

The infant has poor peripheral perfusion, has thready pulses, and continues to show evidence of shock.

Preparation and Administration

The preparation (and administration) of dopamine is very different from that of the medications discussed earlier in this lesson. Dopamine, as you have learned, is administered only as a continuous infusion. Therefore, an intravenous solution containing dopamine must be prepared.

The concentration of the solution prepared will vary based on the:

- Dosage desired,
- Infant's weight, and
- Volume of fluid considered desirable or safe to administer.

A formula that considers these factors has been developed for preparing a dopamine solution. But first you need to know the recommended dosage and how a dopamine dosage is expressed.

Dosage

Begin at 5 mcg/kg/min
(May increase up to 20 mcg/kg/min if necessary)

Since dopamine is given as a continuous infusion, **the dosage is *always* expressed as the *amount of dopamine* to be infused *per kilogram per minute,*** e.g., *5 mcg/kg/min, not* 5 mcg/kg or 5 mcg.

Preparing Solution

A formula commonly used follows:

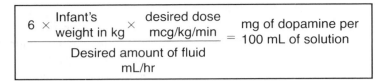

$$\frac{6 \times \frac{\text{Infant's}}{\text{weight in kg}} \times \frac{\text{desired dose}}{\text{mcg/kg/min}}}{\text{Desired amount of fluid mL/hr}} = \frac{\text{mg of dopamine per}}{100 \text{ mL of solution}}$$

Multiply 6 times the infant's weight in *kg* times the desired dose in *mcg/kg/min,* divided by the desired amount of fluid to infuse in *mL/hr* provides you with:

- **the amount of dopamine in mg to add to each 100 mL of solution prepared.**

Infusing Solution

Infusing the solution at the desired mL/hr provides the infant with the desired dose/minute. Remember that an infusion pump must always be used to ensure a controlled infusion rate.

Be sure to clear the dead space in the I.V. tubing. Because the infusion rates, in terms of cc/minute, are relatively slow, it may take some time before the infant actually begins receiving dopamine if the dead space is not cleared first.

Effects

- Strengthens cardiac contractions
- Increases cardiac output
- Raises blood pressure

Anticipated Signs

- Blood pressure should rise.
- Heart rate should stabilize; tachycardia is often present.

Initially increase the infusion rate to 8 mcg/kg/min if the heart rate and blood pressure do not respond as indicated. With consultation you may be advised to increase the infusion rate even more.

Follow-up

First 15 minutes:
- Check the heart rate every 30–60 seconds;
- Check blood pressure every 2 minutes.

After 15 minutes:
- Check heart rate and blood pressure at least every 5 minutes until the blood pressure is stabilized.

The administration of a dopamine drip may need to be continued for several hours. As you attempt to decrease the infusion, be sure that the heart rate and blood pressure stay within a normal range.

Caution:

If an infant has an insufficient response to 20 mcg/kg/min of dopamine, it is highly unlikely that raising the dose further will make a difference. In these circumstances a continuous drip of epinephrine at 0.1 mcg/kg/min may need to be administered.

Example of Dopamine Calculations

Let's apply the formula for preparing the appropriate concentration of dopamine.

- patient's weight = 1200 gm (1.2 kg)
- desired dose = 5 mcg/kg/minute
- desired amount of fluid = 3 mL/hr

$$\frac{6 \times 1.2\ kg \times 5\ mcg/kg/min}{3\ mL/hr} = \begin{array}{l} 12\ mg\ of\ dopamine \\ for\ each\ 100\ mL\ prepared \end{array}$$

Since only 3 mL/hr will be infused, you need to prepare no more than 100 mL of solution. You add 12 mg of dopamine to 100 mL and infuse the solution at a rate of 3 mL/hr. This will provide the infant with a dopamine dosage of 5 mcg/kg/min.

Practice:

For practice, calculate preparing an infusion.

- weight = 3500 gm (3.5 kg)
- desired dose = 8 mcg/kg/min
- desired amount of fluid = 5 mL/hr

How would you prepare the solution?

A. How many mg of dopamine do you need to add if preparing 100 mL? _____

B. How many mg if you are preparing 200 mL? _____

C. How fast would you run the infusion? _____

D. What dose would the infant receive? _____

Answers:

Here are the answers and calculations for the above problems.

$$\frac{6 \times 3.5 \text{ kg} \times 8 \text{ mcg/kg/min}}{5 \text{ mL/hr}}$$

$$\frac{6 \times 3.5 \times 8}{5} = \frac{168}{5} = 33.6 \text{ mg of dopamine per } 100 \text{ mL of solution}$$

A. Add 33.6 mg of dopamine to 100 mL of solution
B. Add 67.2 mg of dopamine to 200 mL of solution
C. Run infusion at 5 mL/hr
D. Dosage received by infant would be 8 mcg/kg/min

Summary

A review of the important information presented about dopamine is presented below.

Indication

During a prolonged resuscitation, dopamine is indicated in a neonate who has received:

- Epinephrine,
- Volume expander, and
- Sodium bicarbonate,

and who has:

- Poor peripheral perfusion, a thready pulse, and continuing evidence of shock.

Dosage

Begin at 5 mcg/kg/min.
(May be necessary to increase to 20 mcg/kg/min.)

Preparation

An intravenous solution for infusion can be prepared using the following formula.

$$\frac{6 \times \text{Infant's weight in kg} \times \text{desired dose mcg/kg/min}}{\text{Desired amount of fluid mL/hr}} = \text{mg of dopamine per } 100 \text{ mL of solution}$$

Administration

Administer as a continuous infusion, using an infusion pump to carefully control flow rate.

Monitor Patient

First 15 minutes:

Every 30–60 seconds—check heart rate,
Every 2 minutes—check blood pressure.

After 15 minutes:

Every 5 minutes—check heart rate *and* blood pressure until the blood pressure is stabilized.

Appendix C: Medications for Neonatal Resuscitation

Medication	Concentration to Administer	Preparation	Dosage/ Route*	Total Dose/Infant		Rate/Precautions
Epinephrine	1:10,000	1 mL	0.1–0.3 mL/kg I.V. or E.T.	**weight** 1 kg 2 kg 3 kg 4 kg	**total mL's** 0.1–0.3 mL 0.2–0.6 mL 0.3–0.9 mL 0.4–1.2 mL	Give rapidly
Volume Expanders	Whole Blood 5% Albumin Normal Saline Ringer's Lactate	40 mL	10 mL/kg I.V.	**weight** 1 kg 2 kg 3 kg 4 kg	**total mL's** 10 mL 20 mL 30 mL 40 mL	Give over 5–10 min
Sodium Bicarbonate	0.5 mEq/mL (4.2% solution)	20 mL or two 10-mL prefilled syringes	2 mEq/kg I.V.	**weight** **total dose** 1 kg 2 mEq 2 kg 4 mEq 3 kg 6 mEq 4 kg 8 mEq	**total mL's** 4 mL 8 mL 12 mL 16 mL	Give *slowly*, over at least 2 min Give only if infant being effectively ventilated
Naloxone	0.4 mg/mL	1 mL	0.1 mg/kg (0.25 mL/kg) I.V., E.T., I.M., S.Q.	**weight** **total dose** 1 kg 0.1 mg 2 kg 0.2 mg 3 kg 0.3 mg 4 kg 0.4 mg	**total mL's** 0.25 mL 0.50 mL 0.75 mL 1.00 mL	Give rapidly I.V., E.T. preferred I.M., S.Q. acceptable
	1.0 mg/mL	1 mL	0.1 mg/kg (0.1 mL/kg) I.V., E.T., I.M., S.Q.	**weight** 1 kg 0.1 mg 2 kg 0.2 mg 3 kg 0.3 mg 4 kg 0.4 mg	0.1 mL 0.2 mL 0.3 mL 0.4 mL	
Dopamine	$6 \times \dfrac{\text{weight} \times \text{desired dose}}{\text{desired fluid (mL/hr)}} = \dfrac{\text{mg of dopamine per 100 mL of solution}}{}$ (kg) (mcg/kg/min)		Begin at 5 mcg/kg/min (may increase to 20 mcg/kg/min if necessary) I.V.	**weight** 1 kg 2 kg 3 kg 4 kg	**total mcg/min** 5–20 mcg/min 10–40 mcg/min 15–60 mcg/min 20–80 mcg/min	Give as a continuous infusion using an infusion pump Monitor HR and BP closely Seek consultation

*I.M. — Intramuscular; E.T. — Endotracheal; I.V. — Intravenous; S.Q. — Subcutaneous

4739.

4739.